STUDY GUIDE for

PATHOPHYSIOLOGY for the HEALTH PROFESSIONS

Third Edition

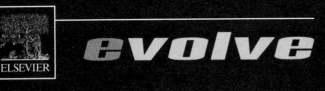

To access your Student Resources, visit:

http://evolve.elsevier.com/Gould/pathophysiology/

Evolve Resources for *Gould: Pathophysiology for the Health Professions*, **3rd Edition**, offers the following features:

Student Resources

- **Challenge Assignments**
  Helpful for student self-evaluation. Assignments involve medical history, sample drug orders, genetics, and research.

- **Quickie Timed Tests**
  Short tests on appendices and miscellaneous topics. Includes suggested time limit.

- **Test Bank**
  This is the same test bank that is provided on the student CD at the back of the textbook.

- **Case Studies**
  These are in addition to those provided on the student CD at the back of the textbook.

- **Lists of Herbal Remedies and Additional Disorders**
  Also provided on the student CD at the back of the textbook, this resource includes brief significant facts for the Additional Disorders.

- **Weblinks**
  Links to places of interest on the web specific to pathophysiology.

- **Content Updates**
  Find out the latest information on relevant issues in the field of pathophysiology.

STUDY GUIDE for

PATHOPHYSIOLOGY for the HEALTH PROFESSIONS

Third Edition

Gwen Buttle, RN, BScN, MEd
Professor
Centre for Health Sciences and International Denturists Education Centre
George Brown College
Toronto, Ontario, Canada

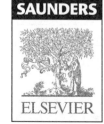

SAUNDERS

ELSEVIER

SAUNDERS
ELSEVIER

1600 John F. Kennedy Blvd.
Ste 1800
Philadelphia, PA 19103-2899

STUDY GUIDE FOR PATHOPHYSIOLOGY FOR THE HEALTH
PROFESSIONS, ED 3

ISBN-13: 978-1-4160-2582-5
ISBN-10: 1-4160-2582-0

Copyright © 2006 by Elsevier Inc.

Notice

Pathophysiology is an ever-changing field. As new research and experience broaden our knowledge, changes in practice, treatment and drug therapy may become necessary or appropriate. Readers are advised to check the most current information provided (i) on procedures featured or (ii) by the manufacturer of each product to be administered, to verify the recommended dose or formula, the method and duration of administration, and contraindications. It is the responsibility of the practitioner, relying on their own experience and knowledge of the patient, to make diagnoses, to determine dosages and the best treatment for each individual patient, and to take all appropriate safety precautions. To the fullest extent of the law, neither the Publisher nor the Author assume any liability for any injury and/or damage to persons or property arising out or related to any use of the material contained in this book.

The Publisher

ISBN-13: 978-1-4160-2582-5
ISBN-10: 1-4160-2582-0

Managing Editor: Mindy Hutchinson
Senior Developmental Editor: Melissa K. Boyle
Publishing Services Manager: Julie Eddy
Project Manager: Andrea Campbell
Design Manager: Teresa McBryan

Printed in the United States of America

Last digit is the print number: 9 8 7 6 5 4 3 2 1

Contents

1 Introduction to Pathophysiology

1. Cells adapt to environmental changes by changing their size, number, and type. For each of the following scenarios, identify the appropriate **adaptive cellular change** or changes that occur, using the following terms:

atrophy	metaplasia
hypertrophy	dysplasia
hyperplasia	neoplasia

   i. the development of callus on the hands of an individual involved in heavy physical labor:

   ii. breast enlargement at puberty:

   iii. a decrease in the size of a leg after being in a cast for 6 weeks:

   iv. the response of skeletal muscle to consistent weight training:

   v. the myocardium in response to prolonged elevated blood pressure:

   vi. the changes that occur in the lower extremities of someone paralyzed below the waist:

   vii. a pressure area under a poorly fitting denture:

   viii. enlargement of the prostate gland with age:

   ix. the response of skeletal muscle to anabolic steroids:

   x. skin changes that occur on the feet and legs of an individual with poorly controlled or undiagnosed diabetes mellitus:

   xi. the changes that often occur over years in the respiratory tract of a smoker:

   xii. the changes responsible for an abnormal Pap smear:

   xiii. the response of the skeletal system to excessive growth hormone:

   xiv. the thyroid gland's response to hypersecretion of thyroid-stimulating hormone:

1

xv. the effect of decreased pituitary gland function on the adrenal glands:

xvi. the liver's response to prolonged drug intoxication (e.g., chronic alcohol abuse):

xvii. the response of the mandible to excessive growth hormone:

xviii. the changes that occur in the urinary bladder when the outflow of urine is obstructed (as might occur with an enlarged prostate gland):

xix. the thyroid gland's response to decreased iodine intake:

xx. the changes that occur in the gallbladder with the development of gallstones:

2. Which cellular adaptation is considered to be the **most dangerous**? Explain why.

3. Define **anaplasia**. Explain the **significance** of anaplasia.

4. List seven causes of cellular damage.
   i.

   ii.

   iii.

   iv.

   v.

   vi.

   vii.

5. Complete the following crossword puzzle:

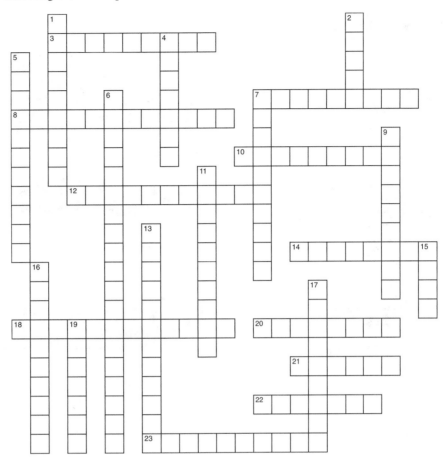

ACROSS
3. a tumor
7. number of new cases of a disease
8. worsening of disease
10. death rate
12. tissue enlargement caused by an increase in cell number
14. cell death
18. development of a disease
20. cause of a disease
21. a specific local change in tissue
22. condition that continues for a prolonged period
23. originating inside the body

DOWN
1. cells that have failed to develop specialized features
2. condition with sudden onset and severe symptoms
4. subjective response to illness
5. tissue enlargement due to increased cell size (two words)
6. risk factor
7. unknown cause
9. deranged cell growth
11. disease caused by a treatment procedure
13. contagious condition
15. an objective indicator of disease
16. substitution of one mature cell type with a different cell type
17. originating outside the body
19. decreased O_2

6. Identify the following cellular adaptations:

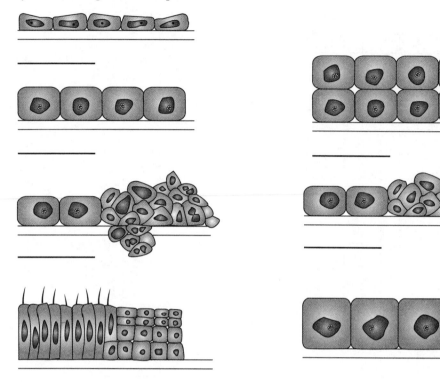

_____

_____

_____   _____

_____   _____

_____   _____

2 Inflammation and Healing

1. What is the body's **first "line of defense"**?

2. Identify the body's **second and third "lines of defense."**

3. Which of the defenses identified above are specific? Explain what is meant by the term "specific."

4. Define **phagocytosis**. Identify types of cells that are phagocytic and where these cells are located within the body.

5. Identify the events of the **"vascular response"** that occur during an inflammatory response. Explain why each change occurs, as well as the consequences of each event.

6. Identify the **five cardinal signs** of an inflammatory response and the cause of each.

7. Outline the events of the **cellular response of an inflammation** in the correct chronological order.

8. Match each of the following terms with the appropriate definition.

   a) involved in cell-mediated immunity

   b) elevated during allergic responses

   c) secrete histamine

   d) the first cells to emigrate to an injured area

   e) involved in antibody production

   f) elevated during chronic inflammations

   g) a source of macrophages

   h) phagocytize microorganisms

   i) **neutrophils** _____

   ii) **basophils** _____

   iii) **eosinophils** _____

   iv) **macrophages** _____

   v) **mast cells** _____

   vi) **monocytes** _____

   vii) **T lymphocytes** _____

   viii) **B lymphocytes** _____

5

9. List the **systemic effects of inflammation**, identifying the reason that each of these manifestations occurs.

10. Compare and contrast **acute and chronic inflammation**, using the following chart:

Characteristic	Acute Inflammation	Chronic Inflammation
Causative agents		
Onset of symptoms		
Intensity of symptoms		
Duration		
Cells involved		
Outcome		

11. The acronym **RICE** is sometimes useful in remembering interventions that can be used to treat inflammation, particularly those caused by athletic injuries:

R–rest

I–ice

C–compression

E–elevation

Explain the rationale for each of these interventions.

12. Identify additional **nonpharmacologic interventions** that could be used to treat inflammation, particularly conditions that are chronic, such as arthritis.

13. State five differences between **nonsteroidal anti-inflammatory drugs (NSAIDs)** and **glucocorticoids or steroidal anti-inflammatory drugs**.

14. Identify differences between **NSAIDs and acetaminophen.**

15. Differentiate between the processes of **resolution and regeneration.** What factors determine which of these processes will occur following an injury?

16. Many factors influence **tissue healing**. Explain how the following factors could complicate or delay healing, stating at least one example to illustrate each one:

   i. the nature of the tissue/location of the wound:

   ii. the nutritional status of the injured individual:

   iii. the size and shape of the wound:

   iv. the drugs that the injured individual is taking:

   v. the age of the individual:

Chapter 2 Inflammation and Healing

vi. the presence of foreign material in the wound:

vii. the blood supply of the injured tissue:

viii. the presence of infection in the damaged tissue:

ix. the degree of immobilization of the injured tissue:

x. pre-existing disease states that exist in the injured individual:

17. Identify potential **complications** that may occur during an inflammatory process and subsequent healing.

18. Describe the **classifications of burns** based on:

i. body surface area:

ii. depth of tissue damage:

19. Explain why full-thickness burns initially may be painless.

20. Define the following terms:

i. **keloid:**

ii. **eschar:**

iii. **stenosis:**

iv. **adhesion:**

v. **ulcer:**

vi. **exudate:**

vii. **contracture:**

3 Immunity and Abnormal Responses

1. State three differences between **inflammation and immunity**.

2. What is a **cell surface antigen**? Why is it important?

3. What are human leukocyte antigens or HLAs? What is the major histocompatibility complex (MHC)?

4. Chemical mediators play an important role in both inflammation and immunity. Identify the source and effects of the major chemical mediators, using the following chart:

Chemical Mediator	Source	Effects
Histamine		
Prostaglandins		
Cytokines (lymphokines, monokines, interleukins, interferon)		
Leukotrienes		
Kinins (bradykinin)		
Complement		

5. Several of the **chemical mediators** have overlapping effects. Identify which ones are responsible for each of the following cellular or body responses:

    i. vasodilation:

    ii. increased capillary permeability:

    iii. chemotaxis:

    iv. pain:

    v. contraction of bronchiolar walls/bronchospasm:

    vi. proliferation of leukocytes:

    vii. pruritus:

    viii. fever:

6. All of the following cells are involved in immunity. Identify the role of each:

Cell Type	Function
Macrophages	
Natural killer (NK) cells	
T-lymphocytes	
Cytotoxic or killer T cells	
Helper T cells (T4 or CD4)	

Cell Type, cont'd	Function, cont'd
Memory T cells	
Suppressor T cells (T8)	
B-lymphocytes	
Plasma cells	
B memory cells	

7. Which type or types of cells play a role in **both** inflammation and immunity?

8. Which cells participate in **both** cellular and humoral immunity?

9. List the five **classes of antibodies or immunoglobulins**, and state the functions of each.

10. Explain how antibodies exert their effects.

11. What is the time frame between exposure to an antigen and the appearance of immunoglobulins in the serum?

12. What is the average length of time required to acquire an **effective antibody titer** following exposure to an antigen?

13. Explain the rationale for "boosters"?

14. Explain why individuals may contract infections such as colds, influenza, and sexually transmitted diseases (STDs) repeatedly.

15. Compare and contrast active and passive immunity using the following chart:

Characteristic	Active Immunity	Passive Immunity
Method of acquiring		
Onset of immunity		
Duration of effectiveness		
Examples		

16. A serious complication of organ transplantation is **organ rejection**. Identify measures that are taken in the attempt to prevent this from happening.

17. A common adverse effect of immunosuppressant drugs is the development of **"opportunistic infections."** What is meant by the term "opportunistic"? Explain why this complication occurs.

18. What medications are often prescribed prophylactically for an individual who is taking immunosuppressant drugs? Explain the rationale.

19. Compare and contrast the different **types of hypersensitivity** reactions, using the following chart:

Type	Mechanism	Effects	Example
I			
II			
III			
IV			

20. Hypovolemic shock is a potential complication of extensive burns (see Chapter 2). Compare and contrast this type of shock with anaphylactic shock using the following chart:

	Hypovolemic Shock	Anaphylactic Shock
Etiology		
Distinguishing features		
Specific treatment		

21. List the types of medications that might be prescribed in the **treatment of allergic conditions**.

13

AUTOIMMUNITY

22. State the underlying mechanism responsible for **autoimmune disorders**.

23. What types of **medications** might be prescribed in the treatment of autoimmune disorders? Explain the rationale for each drug group.

24. How is **systemic lupus erythematosus** diagnosed?

25. Systemic lupus erythematosus has widespread effects virtually throughout the body. Identify common manifestations under the following headings:

    i. skin:

    ii. joints:

    iii. heart:

    iv. blood vessels:

    v. blood:

    vi. kidneys:

    vii. lungs:

    viii. central nervous system:

26. Outline **therapeutic interventions** used in the treatment of lupus erythematosus.

IMMUNODEFICIENCY

27. List common causes of **immunodeficiency**.

28. Identify the **general effects of immunodeficiency**.

29. Identify the types of **medications** that are often prescribed for the immunodeficient individual or immunocompromised host, and explain the rationale for each drug group.

HIV AND AIDS

30. What is the **causative agent** responsible for **HIV and AIDS**? Describe its properties.

31. List the **routes of transmission** of HIV.

32. Identify individuals who are at **high risk** for contracting HIV.

33. What is the usual **incubation period** for HIV? State the possible **range**.

34. How is a **diagnosis of HIV infection** confirmed? What is meant by the **"window period"**?

35. What is the average length of time between infection with HIV and development of **full-blown AIDS**?

36. How is a **diagnosis of AIDS** confirmed?

37. Which cells are targeted by HIV? Identify the consequences of this.

38. Identify possible manifestations of the **initial phase of HIV** infection.

39. As HIV progresses and the individual's immune system becomes more compromised, literally every bodily system is affected. Describe these complications under the following headings:

    i. generalized effects:

    ii. opportunistic infections:

    iii. gastrointestinal manifestations:

    iv. oral manifestations:

    v. respiratory manifestations:

    vi. nervous system manifestations:

    vii. malignancies:

40. Identify **medications** that are used in the treatment of an individual with HIV and AIDS, including those that are prescribed to prevent potential complications.

41. What is the **prognosis** for an individual infected with HIV?

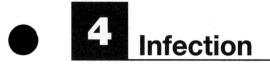 **Infection**

1. Explain the difference between an **inflammation** and an **infection**.

BACTERIA

2. Identify the three **major groups or classifications of bacteria**, including examples of each.

3. Describe the **basic structure** of a bacterium.

4. Some bacteria secrete toxins. Explain the differences between **exotoxins and endotoxins**.

5. What is an **endospore or bacterial spore**? Describe the process of spore formation. Identify bacteria that produce spores.

6. Bacteria reproduce by a process called **binary fission**. Describe this process.

7. Bacterial cells differ from human cells in a number of significant ways. Compare and contrast bacterial and human cells, using the following chart:

	Bacterial Cells	**Human Cells**
Cell wall		
Cell membrane		
Capsule or slime coat		
Flagella		

	Bacterial Cells	Human Cells
Pili or fimbriae		
Cilia		
Membrane-bound organelles (mitochondria, lysosomes, endoplasmic reticulum)		
Ribosomes		
Nucleus		
Number of chromosomes		
Method of reproduction		

VIRUSES

8. Why are viruses said to be **"obligate intracellular parasites"**?

9. Describe the **structure** of a viral particle or virion.

10. Outline the process of **viral replication**.

FUNGI

11. Describe the structure of a fungus.

12. Compare and contrast bacteria, fungi, and viruses, using the following chart:

	Bacteria	Fungus	Virus
Structure			
Method of reproduction			
Method of culturing			
Drugs used to treat			

OTHER MICROORGANISMS

13. List several pathological conditions caused by each of the following types of organisms:

  i. **chlamydiae**:

  ii. **rickettsiae**:

  iii. **mycoplasmas**:

  iv. **protozoa**:

14. What is a **helminth**?

15. What is meant by the term "normal flora" or "resident flora"?

16. Identify areas of the body that lack resident flora and therefore should be sterile.

17. Define the terms **virulence** and **pathogenicity**. Identify factors that increase the virulence and pathogenicity of microorganisms.

CONSOLIDATION OF MICROBIOLOGY

18. Identify the causative agent or agents for each of the following infections. Use the choices listed below.

bacteria	rickettsiae
viruses	chlamydia
fungi	protozoa

   i. pneumocystis carinii pneumonia:

  ii. candidiasis:

 iii. syphilis:

 iv. trichomoniasis:

   v. tuberculosis:

  vi. pneumonia:

 vii. tetanus:

viii. Rocky Mountain spotted fever:

  ix. tinea pedis:

   x. herpes simplex:

  xi. influenza:

 xii. botulism:

INFECTION

19. What is meant by the **"infectious cycle"**? Identify its components and ways in which the cycle can be broken.

20. What is meant by the term **"culture and sensitivity"**?

21. How do the **manifestations** of an infection differ from those of an inflammation?

22. Define the following terms related to **antibacterial drugs**:

    i. antibacterial spectrum:

    ii. bacterial resistance:

    iii. bactericidal:

    iv. bacteriostatic:

23. Explain why it has been difficult to develop **antiviral drugs**.

24. What is probably the **most serious adverse effect** associated with antibacterial drugs?

25. Explain what is meant by the term **superinfection**. What type of microorganism often causes superinfections? Explain why this happens.

26. What is the difference between a superinfection and an **opportunistic infection**?

27. When is it appropriate for a physician to prescribe a **narrow spectrum antibacterial** drug?

28. If an antibacterial drug is bacteriostatic rather than bactericidal, how does the individual ever eliminate the infecting microorganism from his or her body?

29. When would the prescription of a bacteriostatic drug not be advisable?

30. Explain how the **misuse or overuse** of antibacterial agents could lead to the development of bacterial resistance.

31. If antibacterial drugs are not effective in the treatment of viral infections, why are they often prescribed for individuals with chronic viral infections such as hepatitis B, hepatitis C, or HIV?

32. Identify guidelines that an individual should follow to **maximize the effects** of antibacterial medications.

5 Neoplasms

1. Define the following terms:

    i. neoplasm:

    ii. benign:

    iii. malignant:

    iv. carcinoma:

    v. sarcoma:

    vi. anaplasia:

2. Identify the correct name for both benign and malignant tumors in the following locations:

	Benign Tumor	Malignant Tumor
Pancreas		
Fat		
Bone		
Liver		
Cartilage		
Skin		

3. Compare and contrast benign and malignant tumors using the following chart:

	Benign Tumors	Malignant Tumors
Cell growth		
▪ Shape		
▪ Size		
▪ Nucleus		
▪ Differentiation		
▪ Mitosis		
▪ Cell proficiency		
▪ Antigenic properties		
▪ Cohesiveness		
Growth rate		
Presence of capsule		
Spread		
Systemic effects		
Life-threatening		

4. A tumor is a space-occupying mass that produces predictable local effects as it enlarges. Describe the **consequences and manifestations** that could result from the listed effects:

    i. compression of blood vessels:

    ii. compression or obstruction of a tube or duct:

    iii. compression of nerves:

    iv. erosion of blood vessels and other structures:

    v. invasion and replacement of normal tissue:

5. Malignant tumors also have **generalized systemic effects**. Outline the factors that contribute to the development of the following systemic manifestations:

    i. weight loss and cachexia:

    ii. anemia:

    iii. systemic infections:

    iv. bleeding:

6. What is a **paraneoplastic syndrome**?

7. Identify the warning signs of cancer.

8. Explain how each of the following assessment tools could assist in the detection and diagnosis of cancer:

    i. medical history:

    ii. physical examination:

    iii. x-ray, ultrasound, magnetic resonance imaging (MRI), and computed tomography (CT or CAT scan):

iv. tumor markers:

v. biopsy and histological and cytological examinations:

9. Describe how malignant cells **spread** from the original tumor to distant sites in the body. What is this called?

10. Distinguish between the **grading** and **staging** of neoplasms.

11. Differentiate between an **initiating factor** and a **promoter** in relation to carcinogenesis.

12. Identify eight **risk factors** for developing cancer and at least one example of each.

13. Identify the three conventional **interventions** employed in the treatment of cancer. Why are they often used in combination, rather than singly?

14. Treatment for cancer may be **curative, palliative**, or **prophylactic**. Differentiate among these, including an example of each type of treatment.

15. Explain how **radiotherapy** is effective in treating some types of cancer.

16. Identify the mechanisms of action of **antineoplastic medications**.

17. Identify **adverse effects** that commonly occur during both radiotherapy and chemotherapy, and explain why they happen.

18. What is a **biologic response modifier**? How are these agents useful in the treatment of some types of cancer?

19. Outline why **glucocorticoids** may be prescribed during the treatment of cancer.

20. Identify **other types of drugs** that may be used in the treatment of cancer, including the rationale for each.

21. What is the most common form of **skin cancer**?

22. Explain why individuals who have incompetent immune systems are at a higher risk of developing malignancies.

23. Complete the following crossword puzzle:

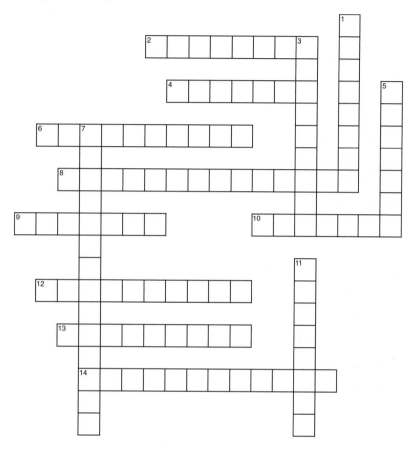

ACROSS
2. severe tissue wasting
4. malignant tumor arising from connective tissue
6. spread of cancer to a distant site
8. transformation of normal cells into cancer cells
9. pre-invasive tumor (hyphenated)
10. degree of differentiation of malignant cells
12. cancer causing agent
13. malignant tumor arising in epithelial tissue
14. invasion

DOWN
1. agents capable of causing alterations in DNA
3. failure of cells to develop specialized features
5. spread of cancer via body secretions
7. conversion of normal cells to cancerous cells
11. the study of cancer

6 Fluid, Electrolyte, and Acid-Base Imbalances

EDEMA

1. Define **edema**.

2. Identify the four **general causes** of edema, and explain how each one results in accumulation of fluid in the extracellular compartment.

3. For each of the following examples, state which of the causes identified in the previous question is responsible for edema formation:

   i. a swollen arm following mastectomy (surgical removal of a breast):

   ii. the abdominal swelling that accompanies liver failure (cirrhosis):

   iii. the swelling that accompanies inflammation:

   iv. the generalized edema that occurs in severe kidney disease:

   v. swelling of the ankles that often happens at the end of the day or after prolonged standing:

   vi. swelling that occurs following multiple tooth extractions:

   vii. edema that may accompany cancer:

   viii. edema that accompanies burns:

   ix. edematous hands and ankles that sometimes accompany excessive ingestion of salt:

   x. the abdominal swelling that occurs with starvation:

   xi. swelling of the ankles associated with heart problems:

   xii. swelling associated with allergic reactions, such as hives:

4. The particular intervention used to treat edema depends on the specific cause. Identify the **type of medication** that could be used to treat the edema in the following scenarios:

    i. swelling of the ankles associated with heart problems:

    ii. after the extraction of four "wisdom teeth":

    iii. a swollen ankle caused by an athletic injury:

    iv. nasal congestion due to allergies:

    v. laryngeal edema caused by an anaphylactic reaction:

    vi. swollen tonsils caused by a streptococcal infection:

5. Identify at least eight **effects of edema**.

DEHYDRATION

6. List eight **causes** of dehydration.

7. Describe the **manifestations** of dehydration. What is the **most serious complication** of dehydration?

8. Identify the **compensatory mechanisms** that would be recruited during dehydration.

ELECTROLYTE IMBALANCES

9. Identify the **electrolyte imbalance** or imbalances that could develop in each of the following situations:

    i. renal failure:

    ii. prolonged vomiting:

    iii. insufficient secretion of antidiuretic hormone:

    iv. prolonged use of corticosteroids:

    v. hyperparathyroidism:

vi. excessive sweating:

vii. prolonged immobility:

viii. diuretic therapy:

ix. aldosterone insufficiency:

x. inadequate dietary intake of vitamin D:

xi. cancers involving bone:

xii. prolonged diarrhea:

10. Define **tetany**. Identify the electrolyte imbalance in which tetany occurs.

11. Identify the electrolyte imbalances that affect normal **cardiac function**.

12. What electrolyte imbalance may result in the formation of **kidney stones**?

ACID BASE

13. Explain the difference between a **volatile and nonvolatile acid**.

14. State the normal **bicarbonate ion to carbonic acid ratio**.

15. Identify the **four major buffer systems**.

16. An individual's bicarbonate:carbonic acid ratio is 10:1. What acid-base imbalance is present? What manifestations would the individual experience?

17. For each of the following scenarios, identify which acid-base imbalance could potentially develop. Also identify the compensatory mechanism(s) that might prevent this from occurring:

    i. prolonged corticosteroid therapy:

    ii. chronic bronchitis:

iii. induced vomiting (e.g., bulimia):

iv. narcotic or barbiturate overdose resulting in respiratory depression:

v. fasting:

vi. panic attack with hyperventilation:

vii. pneumonia, with severe bronchial congestion:

viii. hyperaldosteronism:

ix. chronic diarrhea:

x. uncontrolled diabetes mellitus

xi. renal failure:

7 Congenital and Genetic Disorders

1. Explain the difference between an **inherited disorder** and a **developmental disorder**.

2. Define **teratogenesis**. Identify at least six **teratogenic agents**.

3. Explain how poor **maternal nutrition** during pregnancy might cause a developmental disorder. Identify several examples.

4. Explain how **labor and delivery** of a child could be responsible for a congenital disorder.

5. Differentiate between an **inherited disorder** and a **chromosomal disorder**.

6. Outline the etiology of **chromosomal disorders**.

7. Define each of the following terms and then draw a diagram to illustrate how each could occur:

   i. **monosomy**:

   ii. **trisomy**:

8. What appears to be a significant **risk factor** for chromosomal disorders?

9. Explain what is meant by a **"multifactorial disorder."** Identify several examples.

10. Explain the difference between the **carrier** of an infectious disease such as hepatitis B and the carrier of a genetic disorder.

11. In what type or types of inherited disorders is there a **carrier** state?

12. What is the genotype of a carrier, heterozygous or homozygous? Does a carrier of a genetic disorder usually become symptomatic?

13. Let "H" represent an **autosomal dominant disorder**. Complete the following Punnett square, and then answer the accompanying questions:

Father

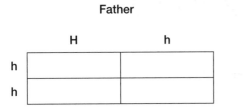

   i. Which parent is affected by this disorder, the father or mother?

   ii. What is the probability that this couple will produce a child with the disorder?

   iii. What is the probability that this couple will produce a child who is a carrier of the disease? Explain.

14. Let "H" represent an **autosomal dominant disorder**. Complete the following Punnett square, and then answer the accompanying questions:

Father

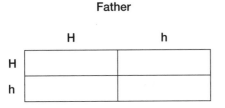

   i. Which parent is affected by this disorder?

   ii. What is the probability that this couple will produce a child with the disease?

15. Let "t" represent an **autosomal recessive disorder**. Complete the following Punnett square, and then answer the accompanying questions:

Father

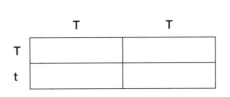

Chapter 7 Congenital and Genetic Disorders

i. Which parent is:
   a) affected by this disorder?

   b) a carrier of this disorder?

   c) asymptomatic in relation to this disorder?

ii. What is the probability that this couple will produce a child:
   a) with the disorder?

   b) who is a carrier of the disorder?

   c) who is phenotypically normal?

   d) who is not a carrier?

16. Let "t" represent an **autosomal recessive disorder**. Complete the following Punnett square, and then answer the accompanying questions:

Father

	T	t
T		
t		

i. Which parent is:
   a) affected by this disorder?

   b) a carrier of this disorder?

   c) asymptomatic in relation to this disorder?

ii. What is the probability that this couple will produce a child:
   a) with the disorder?

   b) who is a carrier of the disorder?

   c) who is phenotypically normal?

   d) who is not a carrier?

17. Let "t" represent an **autosomal recessive disorder**. Complete the following Punnett square, and then answer the accompanying questions:

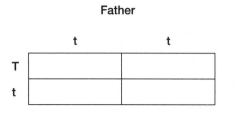

Father

	t	t
T		
t		

    i. Which parent is:
      a) affected by this disorder?

      b) a carrier of this disorder?

      c) asymptomatic in relation to this disorder?

    ii. What is the probability that this couple will produce a child:
      a) with the disorder?

      b) who is a carrier of the disorder?

      c) who is phenotypically normal?

      d) who is not a carrier?

18. A newborn is diagnosed with phenylketonuria (PKU), an autosomal recessive disorder. Neither of his parents have this disease.

    i. What is the baby's genotype?

    ii. Which parent is a carrier of PKU?

    iii. If this couple have a second child, what is the probability that he or she will also have phenylketonuria?

    iv. What is the probability that any of the baby's siblings will be carriers of phenylketonuria?

19. Let "t" represent an **autosomal recessive disorder**. Complete the following Punnett square, and then answer the accompanying questions:

Father

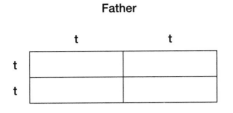

i. Which parent is:
a) affected by this disorder?

b) a carrier of this disorder?

c) asymptomatic in relation to this disorder?

ii. What is the probability that this couple will produce a child:
a) with the disorder?

b) who is a carrier of the disorder?

c) who is phenotypically normal?

d) who is not a carrier?

20. **Sex-linked disorders** are often referred to as "X-linked" because the abnormal gene is usually carried on the X chromosome. Let "H" represent the normal gene and "h" the abnormal one. Complete the following Punnett squares, and then answer the accompanying questions:

Square A

Square B

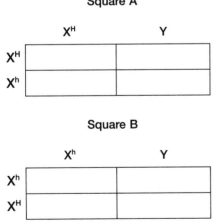

Referring to Square A:

   i. Which parent is:
     a) affected by this disorder?

     b) a carrier of this disorder?

   ii. What is the probability that this couple will produce a child with the disorder?

   iii. What would be the sex of that child?

   iv. What is the probability that this couple will produce a child who is a carrier of this disorder? What would be the sex of that child?

   v. What is the probability of producing a genotypically and phenotypically normal:
     a) son?

     b) daughter?

Referring to Square B:

   i. Which parent is:
     a) affected by this disorder?

     b) a carrier of this disorder?

     c) genotypically and phenotypically normal?

   ii. What is the probability that this couple's:
     a) daughters will be carriers of this disorder?

     b) daughters will be affected by this disorder?

     c) sons will be carriers of this disorder?

     d) sons will be affected by this disorder?

21. How could a female individual have a sex-linked disorder? Draw a Punnett square to illustrate this scenario.

22. A boy is diagnosed with Duchenne's muscular dystrophy, a sex-linked disorder. Neither of his parents have this disease.

    i. What is the child's genotype?

    ii. Which parent is a carrier?

    iii. If this couple have a second child, what is the probability that he or she will also have cystic fibrosis?

    iv. If the child does have a sibling with muscular dystrophy, will it be a brother or sister? Explain.

    v. What is the probability that any of the child's siblings will be carriers of cystic fibrosis? Will the carriers be male or female? Explain.

23. Identify the classification of the following conditions (e.g., autosomal dominant chromosomal, etc.):

    i. colon cancer:

    ii. cystic fibrosis:

    iii. cerebral palsy:

    iv. familial hypercholesterolemia:

    v. Duchenne's muscular dystrophy:

    vi. sickle cell anemia:

    vii. hemophilia A:

    viii. Klinefelter's syndrome:

    ix. phenylketonuria:

    x. Huntington's disease:

    xi. Tay-Sachs disease:

    xii. schizophrenia:

Chapter 7 Congenital and Genetic Disorders

xiii. cleft lip and palate:

xiv. Turner's syndrome:

24. What type of disorder is **Down syndrome**? How can it be diagnosed prenatally? What is the karyotype of an individual with Down syndrome?

25. Outline the abnormalities or problems associated with Down syndrome.

26. Describe the characteristic appearance of an individual with Down syndrome.

8 Diseases Associated with Adolescence

1. Match the following terms with the correct definition:

a) condition characterized by alternating "binge and purge" behavior

i) lordosis _____

b) lateral curvature of the spine

ii) kyphosis _____

c) extreme weight loss caused by self-starvation

iii) scoliosis _____

d) exaggerated concave curvature of the lumbar spine

iv) osteoporosis _____

e) demineralization of bone

v) osteomyelitis _____

f) exaggerated convex curvature of the thoracic spine

vi) anorexia nervosa _____

g) bone infection

vii) bulimia nervosa _____

2. Identify **risk factors** for the development of **osteomyelitis**.

3. Outline the **pathophysiology** of osteomyelitis.

4. Distinguish between **anorexia nervosa** and **bulimia nervosa**.

5. What is the causative agent of **mononucleosis**?

6. List the **manifestations and potential complications** of mononucleosis.

9 The Relationship Between Pregnancy and Disease

1. Match the following terms with the correct definition:

   a) milk production

   b) premature separation of the placenta from the uterine wall

   c) pregnancy

   d) inflammation of uterine lining

   e) severe hypertension which occurs as a complication of pregnancy

   f) number of pregnancies

   g) number of viable pregnancies

   i) **gestation** _____

   ii) **gravidity** _____

   iii) **parity** _____

   iv) **eclampsia** _____

   v) **abruptio placentae** _____

   vi) **lactation** _____

   vii) **endometritis** _____

2. Describe the potential **complications of pregnancy**.

3. Explain why **Rh incompatibility** occurs. Describe the manifestations and complications of Rh incompatibility.

4. What is **RhoGAM**? Explain how its administration prevents an Rh incompatibility.

10 Aging and the Disease Processes

1. Describe the **effects of aging** on the following body systems:

    i. endocrine system:

    ii. reproductive system:

    iii. cardiovascular system:

    iv. musculoskeletal system:

    v. respiratory system:

    vi. nervous system:

    vii. gastrointestinal system:

    viii. urinary system:

2. Explain why the elderly are at a higher risk for both infections and cancer than younger individuals.

3. Match the following terms with the correct definitions:

    a) inability to control urination   i) **atherosclerosis** _____

    b) farsightedness   ii) **cataract** _____

    c) predetermined cell death   iii) **apoptosis** _____

    d) elasticity of the lungs   iv) **glaucoma** _____

    e) excessive urination at night   v) **incontinence** _____

f) opacity of the ocular lens

g) deposition of fat in arterial walls

h) dry mouth

i) increased intraocular pressure

vi) nocturia _____

vii) presbyopia _____

viii) xerostomia _____

ix) compliance _____

11 Effects of Immobility

1. Summarize the **effects of immobility** throughout the body.

2. Match the following terms with the correct definitions:

   a) stationary blood clot

   b) collapse of lung tissue

   c) sudden drop in blood pressure when change in position occurs

   d) floating blood clot

   e) pressure sore or bedsore

   f) paralysis below the waist

   g) joint deformity caused by excessive scarring

   h) paralysis of one side of the body

   i) atelectasis _____

   ii) contracture _____

   iii) decubitus ulcer _____

   iv) embolus _____

   v) hemiplegia _____

   vi) orthostatic hypotension _____

   vii) paraplegia _____

   viii) thrombus _____

12 The Influence of Stress

1. Identify the **hormones** that are secreted during stress, including the source and effects of each one.

2. Summarize the effects of the **sympathetic nervous system** during stress.

3. Explain why prolonged stress, such as that associated with divorce or professional difficulties, can be detrimental to health.

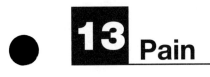

13 Pain

1. List the **causes** of pain.

2. Describe the steps involved in the **perception of pain**, from the stimulus to interpretation. Include all the anatomical structures that are involved in the pathway.

3. What is meant by **referred pain**? Explain why it occurs. Describe an example of referred pain.

4. Outline measures used to **control pain**, including the rationale for each.

5. Identify factors that may influence an individual's **response to pain**.

6. Complete the following chart, which compares and contrasts non-narcotic and narcotic analgesics:

	Non-Narcotic Analgesics	**Narcotic Analgesics**
Action		
Adverse effects		
Uses		
Examples		

7. Identify three common **types of anesthesia**, and state an example of when each would be employed.

14 Substance Abuse

1. Identify substances that are commonly abused.

2. Explain the potential complications of substance abuse.

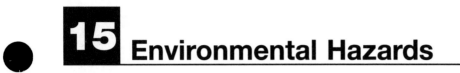
15 Environmental Hazards

1. Identify nine types of environmental hazards, and state an example of each.

16 Introduction to Basic Pharmacology and Selected Therapies

1. Identify the **reasons** for the prescribing of drugs.

2. Distinguish between the **therapeutic effects** and **adverse or side effects** of a drug.

3. Medications may be administered by a number of different routes. Describe what is meant by each of the following drug routes, and state several examples of medications that are commonly taken this way:

  i. **topical**:

  ii. **transdermal**:

  iii. **oral**:

  iv. **sublingual**:

  v. **subcutaneous**:

  vi. **intramuscular**:

  vii. **intravenous**:

  viii. **inhalation**:

4. Drugs are used for both systemic and local effects. Which route of administration is used to achieve a **local effect**?

5. Complete the following chart comparing and contrasting various routes of drug administration:

	Onset of Action	Advantages	Disadvantages
Topical			
Transdermal			
Oral			
Sublingual			
Subcutaneous			
Intramuscular			
Intravenous			
Inhalation			

6. Arrange the routes of drug administration according to rapidity of onset, from the fastest to the slowest.

7. Describe what happens to a drug once it is absorbed into the blood.

8. Explain the manner in which many drugs exert their effects at a cellular level.

9. Where are most drugs **metabolized**? How is this achieved?

10. How are most drugs or their metabolites **excreted** from the body?

11. Explain the ways in which diseases of the liver or kidneys could affect drug activity.

12. Why are individuals with chronic lung disease considered to be at high risk for complications when they receive a general anesthetic?

13. Explain how each of the following factors may influence drug action:

   i. age:

   ii. body weight:

   iii. sex:

   iv. psychological factors/emotional state:

   v. presence of disease (e.g., heart disease, liver disease, kidney disease):

   vi. time of administration (in relation to meals; time of day):

   vii. route of administration:

   viii. drug dosage:

   ix. drug formulation (e.g., liquid, capsule, enteric coated):

   x. client compliance:

   xi. environmental factors (e.g., temperature, odors, noise):

   xii. drug interactions:

14. Define the following terms, and state an example for each:

   i. hypersensitivity reaction:

   ii. idiosyncratic reaction:

   iii. potentiation:

Chapter 16 Introduction to Basic Pharmacology and Selected Therapies

iv. synergistic effect:

v. antagonistic effect:

vi. teratogenic effect:

vii. tolerance:

viii. placebo effect:

15. Differentiate between the **generic** and **chemical names** of a specific drug.

16. Describe each of the following **treatment modalities**:

i. **physiotherapy**:

ii. **speech therapy**:

iii. **occupational therapy**:

iv. **homeopathy**:

v. **osteopathy**:

vi. **aromatherapy**:

17 Blood and Lymphatic Disorders

ERYTHROCYTES

1. Describe the normal **"life cycle"** of an erythrocyte, including where it is produced, its life span, and where and how it is destroyed.

2. State the **normal range** for both **red blood cell (RBC) count and hemoglobin,** differentiating between the values found in males and females.

3. Define **anemia.**

4. List the **general manifestations** for all types of anemias.

5. Complete the following chart comparing and contrasting the different types of anemia:

Type of Anemia	Etiology	Specific Manifestations	Specific Treatment
Iron deficiency anemia			
Pernicious anemia— Vitamin B_{12} deficiency anemia			
Aplastic anemia			
Thalassemia			
Sickle cell anemia			

6. **Sickle cell anemia** is an inherited disorder. What is the pattern of inheritance for this disorder? What is the genotype of an individual with sickle cell anemia?

7. What is meant by the **"sickle cell trait"**? What is the genotype of an individual who has this trait?

8. A woman with sickle cell trait is pregnant with the child of a man who has sickle cell anemia. Draw a Punnett square to illustrate this scenario.

i. What is the probability that the child will have sickle cell anemia?

ii. What is the probability that the child will have sickle cell trait?

iii. What is the probability that the child will have neither sickle cell trait nor disease?

iv. What is the probability that any future child that this couple conceives will have sickle cell anemia?

9. Describe the **pathophysiology** of sickle cell anemia.

10. What precipitates **"sickling"**?

11. What is meant by a **"crisis"**? Identify the potential **complications** of a sickling crisis.

12. Explain why an individual with sickle cell anemia may experience the following **manifestations**:

i. jaundice:

ii. cerebrovascular accident:

iii. frequent infections:

iv. splenomegaly:

v. congestive heart failure:

13. Is there any means of preventing sickle cell anemia?

14. Define **polycythemia**.

15. Differentiate between **primary and secondary polycythemia**.

16. Describe the **manifestations and complications** of polycythemia.

17. Identify three therapeutic interventions used in the **treatment of polycythemia**.

BLOOD CLOTTING

18. Draw a flow chart representing the three steps involved in **blood coagulation**.

19. List the **warning signs** of excessive bleeding.

20. Describe **diagnostic tests** that can be employed to identify and/or monitor bleeding disorders.

21. Identify six **causes of abnormal bleeding**, explaining how each interferes with normal hemostasis.

22. Describe how each of the following factors would affect **hemostasis** (i.e., promote or delay blood clotting), and explain why:

    i. liver disease:

    ii. ingestion of aspirin (ASA):

    iii. prolonged antibiotic therapy:

    iv. administration of heparin:

    v. vitamin K deficiency:

vi. prolonged inactivity (e.g., post-operatively or sitting on a plane for many hours):

vii. polycythemia:

viii. thrombocytopenia:

ix. increased hematocrit:

x. administration of warfarin (Coumadin):

23. **Hemophilia A**, or classic hemophilia, is an inherited disorder. What is the pattern of inheritance for this disorder? What is the genotype of an individual with hemophilia A?

24. A woman is a carrier for hemophilia A. She is pregnant with the child of a man who does not have hemophilia. What is her genotype for this disorder? Draw a Punnett square to illustrate this scenario.

i. What is the probability that the child she is carrying will have hemophilia A? Would a child with hemophilia be a male or female?

ii. What is the probability that the child will be a carrier of hemophilia? What would be the sex of a child who is a carrier?

iii. What is the probability that the child will neither have hemophilia nor be a carrier of the disease?

iv. What is the probability that any future sons whom this couple conceives will have hemophilia?

v. What is the probability that any future daughters whom this couple conceives will be carriers of hemophilia?

25. A man with hemophilia A marries a woman whose father has hemophilia A.

i. What is the man's genotype?

ii. What is his wife's genotype?

Draw a Punnett square to demonstrate this scenario.

    i. What is the probability that any children whom this couple produces will have hemophilia?

    ii. What is the probability that any children whom this couple produces will be carriers of hemophilia?

    iii. What will be the sex of a child who is a carrier?

26. Describe the pathophysiology and manifestations of **disseminated intravascular coagulation**.

LEUKOCYTES

27. Define **leukemia**.

28. What is a "blast" cell? Describe its characteristics.

29. Outline the two **major classifications** of leukemia.

30. Identify individuals who are considered at **high risk** for the development of leukemia.

31. What test could be used to **confirm** a diagnosis of leukemia?

32. The **manifestations** of leukemia are diverse and widespread throughout the body. Complete the following chart, explaining why each of the signs and symptoms occurs:

Manifestation	Rationale
Weight loss and fatigue	
Anemia	

Manifestation, cont'd	Rationale, cont'd
Thrombocytopenia	
Multiple infections, including those caused by microorganisms of low virulence	
Increased bleeding and even severe hemorrhage	
Kidney stones	
Fever	
Lymphadenopathy	
Splenomegaly and hepatomegaly	
Bone pain	

33. Describe the **therapeutic interventions** used in the treatment of leukemia, including the adverse effects or complications of each.

34. Describe the **prognosis** for leukemia.

35. Complete the following chart comparing and contrasting acute and chronic leukemia:

	Acute Leukemia	Chronic Leukemia
Age of onset		
Course of disease		
Severity of symptoms		
Number of blast cells		
Response to treatment		
Prognosis		

LYMPHATIC DISORDERS

36. What type of cell is used to diagnosis **Hodgkin's disease**? Describe this cell.

37. Outline the basis for the **staging** of Hodgkin's disease.

38. Describe the **manifestations** of Hodgkin's, through the four stages.

39. Identify **therapeutic interventions** used in the treatment of Hodgkin's disease.

40. Explain how **non-Hodgkin's lymphoma** differs from Hodgkin's disease.

41. Define **multiple myeloma**.

42. Describe the manifestations of **multiple myeloma**, including the reason that each occurs.

CONSOLIDATION

43. For each of the following characteristics, identify the blood or lymphatic disorder or disorders in which they occur:

   i. diagnosed by presence of Reed Sternberg cell:

   ii. involves both excessive bleeding and clotting:

   iii. decreased or lack of intrinsic factor production:

iv. characterized by primitive blast cells:

v. sex-linked bleeding disorder:

vi. increased production of erythrocytes:

vii. frequent adverse effect of chemotherapy:

viii. may result in impaired growth and development:

ix. common in individuals from the Mediterranean area:

x. may be accompanied by jaundice:

xi. may be accompanied by loss of coordination:

xii. a neoplastic disorder involving the red blood cells:

xiii. more prevalent in individuals with Down syndrome:

xiv. generalized pruritus is common:

xv. predisposes individual to infections:

18 Cardiovascular Disorders

ATHEROSCLEROSIS

1. Identify nine **risk factors** for developing atherosclerosis. Indicate which ones are modifiable and which ones are not. Note that these are the same risk factors for heart disease.

2. Describe the process of **atheroma formation**, from the initial fatty streaks in the intima to a complicated plaque.

3. Describe the significance of plaque formation, including five potential **complications of atherosclerosis**.

4. Which vessels are affected by atherosclerosis?

5. Describe, in detail, the therapeutic interventions used in the treatment of atherosclerosis under the following headings:

   i. Diet:

   ii. Exercise:

   iii. Medications—Explain the rationale for prescribing the following drugs:

      a. antilipidemics or lipid-lowering drugs:

      b. platelet inhibitors:

      c. anticoagulants:

      d. antihypertensives:

   iv. Lifestyle/behavioral modifications—Identify measures that an individual should adopt to stop the progression of atherosclerosis:

v. Surgical Intervention—Describe the following surgical procedures:

a. endarterectomy:

b. angioplasty:

c. coronary artery bypass graft:

HEART

6. Locate and label each of the following structures on the accompanying diagram of the heart:

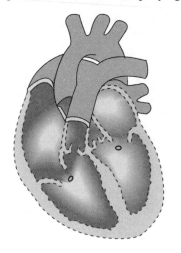

Structures
- right atrium
- left atrium
- right ventricle
- left ventricle
- inferior vena cava
- superior vena cava
- pulmonary artery
- pulmonary veins
- interatrial septum
- interventricular septum
- tricuspid valve
- mitral (bicuspid valve)
- pulmonary semilunar valve
- aortic semilunar valve
- aorta

ANGINA PECTORIS (AP)

7. Define **angina pectoris**.

8. What is the **underlying pathology** involved in angina pectoris?

9. Identify disorders that may **cause** or **predispose** an individual to angina.

10. What is the **most serious complication** of angina pectoris?

11. The factors listed below often **precipitate an attack** (i.e., pain) in an individual with a history of angina. Explain the mechanism involved for each of them:

    i. smoking a cigarette or being exposed to second-hand smoke:

    ii. going from a warm environment into the cold:

    iii. engaging in an argument or other stressful behavior:

    iv. exercise, such as climbing a flight of stairs or rushing to catch a bus:

12. Describe the **classic manifestations** of an **anginal attack**. What is the usual duration of an anginal attack?

13. What type of **drug** is used to treat an **acute anginal attack**? Explain how these drugs relieve chest pain.

14. State a common example of the drug group identified above. How is this drug administered? What is the advantage of this route of administration?

15. Outline the **management of an anginal attack**.

16. When should emergency medical services (EMS) be requested?

17. The drug groups identified in the accompanying chart are often prescribed alone or in combination to control angina and prevent periods of myocardial hypoxia. Explain the action of each type and how each would prevent anginal pain. Also identify adverse effects and one example for each group.

Drug Group	Action and Effects	Adverse Effects	Example
β-adrenergic blockers			
Calcium channel blockers			
Nitrates (vasodilators; transdermal or oral form)			

18. List **other types of medication** that might be prescribed for an individual with angina, and explain the rationale for each.

19. Identify **surgical interventions** that might be used in the treatment of angina.

20. Describe **nonpharmacological interventions** that could help to control angina.

21. A client/patient states that he has angina pectoris. Identify **additional information** that should be obtained from this individual.

22. Identify measures that would help decrease the chance of an individual experiencing an **anginal attack**.

MYOCARDIAL INFARCTION (MI)

23. Define **myocardial infarction**.

24. State three **causes of myocardial infarction**, and indicate which one occurs most frequently.

25. List the **warning signs** of a myocardial infarction.

26. Differentiate between a **transmural and intramural infarction**.

27. What is the **most common site** of an MI?

28. Describe the **pathophysiology** of a myocardial infarction.

29. Describe the **manifestations** of a myocardial infarction.

30. How could a **diagnosis** of myocardial infarction be **confirmed**?

31. What are **serum enzymes**? What is their significance in someone who has suffered a myocardial infarction? Differentiate between enzymes and isoenzymes.

32. Explain why the **electrocardiogram (ECG)** would change after a myocardial infarction.

33. Identify **other diagnostic tools** that could be used to support the diagnosis of MI, and explain the rationale for each.

34. What **complication** of myocardial infarction is responsible for the greatest number of deaths? Why is this complication so serious?

35. Describe **other complications** that may accompany a myocardial infarction.

36. Identify the **therapeutic interventions** used in the treatment of a myocardial infarction, and include the rationale for each.

37. Identify at least four differences between angina pectoris and myocardial infarction.

38. Locate and label the components of the heart's conduction system on the following diagram:

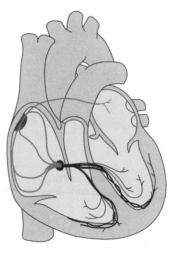

Structures
- sino atrial (SA) node
- atrioventricular (AV) node
- atrioventricular (AV) bundle (bundle of His)
- right bundle branch
- left bundle branch
- Purkinje fibers

39. Outline the path of a **cardiac impulse**.

40. Label the following diagram of an electrocardiogram (ECG):

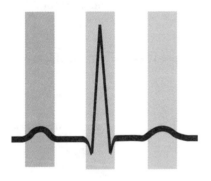

41. Explain what is represented by each segment of the ECG tracing:

    i. P wave:

    ii. QRS complex:

    iii. T wave:

42. Define **arrhythmia** or **dysrhythmia**.

43. List several conditions in which cardiac arrhythmias occur.

44. Match the following terms with the correct definition:

a) heart rate greater than 350 beats per minute

b) extra heartbeat arising in the ventricles

c) heart rate less than 60 beats per minute

d) slowing or no transmission of impulses between atria and ventricles

e) additional heartbeat originating in atria

f) restoration of normal cardiac rhythm by electrical shock

g) heart rate between 160 and 350 beats/minute

h) extra beat originating outside the SA node

i) heart rate between 100 and 160 beats per minute

i) **cardioversion** _____

ii) **bradycardia** _____

iii) **ectopic beat** _____

iv) **flutter** _____

v) **fibrillation** _____

vi) **heart block** _____

vii) **premature atrial contraction (PAC)** _____

viii) **premature ventricular contraction (PVC)** _____

ix) **tachycardia** _____

45. Why is a rapid resting heart rate undesirable?

46. Why is an excessively slow heart rate undesirable?

47. The drug groups identified in the accompanying chart are often prescribed alone or in combination to control arrhythmias. Explain the action of each and how they would control or prevent arrhythmias. Also identify adverse effects and one example for each group.

Chapter 18 Cardiovascular Disorders

Drug Group	Action and Effects	Adverse Effects	Example
β-adrenergic blockers			
Calcium channel blockers			
Digitalis (cardiac glycosides)			

48. An individual who has been diagnosed with cardiac arrhythmias may have a history of atherosclerosis and other heart-related conditions, such as angina or a previous myocardial infarction. Identify other medications that such an individual may be taking to control these conditions.

49. What is an **electronic pacemaker**?

50. Why is it important to know whether a client has a pacemaker?

HEART FAILURE

51. Identify **causes** of congestive heart failure.

52. Describe the **compensatory mechanisms** that are recruited in early heart failure to maintain cardiac output.

53. The consequences of heart failure are often referred to as the **"backward" and "forward"** effects. Explain what is meant by these terms.

54. One side of the heart usually fails first, depending on the specific cause. Complete the following chart comparing and contrasting right-sided and left-sided heart failure:

	Right-Sided Heart Failure	Left-Sided Heart Failure
Cause		
Backward effects		
Forward effects		
Manifestations		

55. Identify the typical **initial symptom** or complaint of:

    i. right-sided heart failure:

    ii. left-sided heart failure:

56. Explain why each of the following **manifestations** occurs with congestive heart failure:

    i. splenomegaly:

    ii. ascites:

    iii. orthopnea:

    iv. cough:

    v. hemoptysis:

    vi. distended neck veins:

    vii. decreased urine output:

viii. nocturia:

ix. polycythemia:

57. Many different **therapeutic interventions** are used in the treatment of congestive heart failure. Explain the rationale for each of the treatment measures listed below:

i. low sodium diet:

ii. low cholesterol diet:

iii. compression stockings:

iv. continuous oxygen therapy:

v. diuretics:

vi. potassium supplement:

vii. angiotensin-converting enzyme (ACE) inhibitors:

viii. digoxin:

ix. platelet inhibitor or anticoagulant:

x. sedative or antianxiety agent:

CONGENITAL HEART DEFECTS

58. List factors that may contribute to the **development** of congenital heart defects.

59. Define the following terms:

i. septal defect:

ii. valvular incompetence:

iii. regurgitation:

iv. prolapse:

v. stenosis:

vi. heart murmur:

60. How are most congenital heart defects **detected**?

61. What are the **consequences** of all significant heart defects?

62. Distinguish between a **"left-to-right shunt"** and a **"right-to-left shunt."** Describe the composition of systemic blood, and explain the implications in each case.

63. Outline the **general manifestations** of a large heart defect.

64. Explain the consequences of a **large ventricular septal defect**, including the complications that develop if the defect is not surgically corrected.

65. To understand the **consequences of a heart valve defect**, it is important to consider what is happening "behind" the valve (the **"backward" effect**), as well as what's happening "in front" of it (the **"forward" effect**). Complete the following chart comparing and contrasting selected valve defects:

Defect	Backward Effects	Forward Effects	Manifestations
Mitral stenosis			
Mitral regurgitation			
Aortic stenosis			

Defect, cont'd	Backward Effects, cont'd	Forward Effects, cont'd	Manifestations, cont'd
Aortic regurgitation			
Pulmonary stenosis			
Pulmonary regurgitation			

66. Identify conditions that are usually associated with **heart murmurs**.

67. Describe the four abnormalities that are present in **tetralogy of Fallot**. Outline the direction of blood flow or draw a diagram to illustrate blood direction. Describe the implications of altered blood flow.

68. Describe **therapeutic interventions** used in the treatment of heart defects.

69. A client states that he previously had a heart murmur but the defective valve was replaced with a prosthetic valve.

   i. What medication will he be taking? Explain the rationale for this drug.

   ii. What medications will he require if he is undergoing an invasive procedure such as tooth scaling (cleaning) or dental surgery? Explain why this is necessary.

RHEUMATIC FEVER, RHEUMATIC HEART DISEASE AND INFECTIVE ENDOCARDITIS

70. What microorganism precipitates rheumatic fever?

71. Identify individuals who are at **high risk** for developing rheumatic fever.

72. Describe the **pathophysiology** of rheumatic fever.

73. Describe the **manifestations** of rheumatic fever under the following headings:

    i. general manifestations of inflammation:

    ii. pericarditis:

    iii. myocarditis:

    iv. endocarditis:

    v. polyarthritis:

    vi. skin manifestations:

    vii. subcutaneous nodules:

    viii. chorea:

74. Which pathological change or effect is considered to be the **most serious**? Explain why.

75. Identify measures used to **diagnose** rheumatic fever.

76. The **treatment of rheumatic fever** involves the use of several different types of drugs. Complete the following chart, identifying the effects of each type of medication as well as providing an example:

Medication	Effects	Example
Antibiotics		
NSAIDs		
Corticosteroids		

Medication, cont'd	Effects, cont'd	Example, cont'd
Antipyretic		
Antiarrhythmics		
Muscle relaxants		

77. Outline **other measures** used in the treatment of rheumatic fever.

78. Distinguish between **rheumatic fever** and **rheumatic heart disease**.

79. Which heart valve is **most commonly affected** by rheumatic heart disease?

80. Why is **ASA** (aspirin) often prescribed for individuals with a history of rheumatic heart disease?

81. Why are individuals with a history of rheumatic heart disease at an **increased risk** of developing **infective endocarditis**?

82. Explain why individuals with a history of rheumatic heart disease require **prophylactic antibiotic coverage** before any invasive procedure, such as dental surgery.

83. Severely damaged heart valves may be surgically replaced with **prosthetic valves**. Explain why someone with a prosthetic heart valve will still be required to take ASA (or some other platelet inhibitor or anticoagulant) for the rest of his or her life and why such a patient will still require antibiotic coverage before invasive procedures.

84. Differentiate between **subacute and acute infective endocarditis** (formerly known as *bacterial endocarditis*). Identify the microbial agents involved in each type.

85. Identify individuals who are at **high risk** for developing each type of infective endocarditis.

86. Outline the **pathophysiology** of infective endocarditis.

87. Describe the **manifestations and complications** of infective endocarditis.

88. How is a **diagnosis** of infective endocarditis confirmed?

89. Describe the **treatment** for infective endocarditis.

90. Complete the following chart comparing and contrasting rheumatic fever and infective endocarditis:

	Rheumatic Fever	Infective Endocarditis
Causative agent(s)		
Predisposing factors		
Manifestations and complications		
Antibiotic of choice		
Prophylactic antibiotic coverage?		

HYPERTENSION

91. Define hypertension. Include numerical values in your definition. How does age affect the criteria for hypertension?

92. Differentiate between **essential** and **secondary** hypertension.

93. List conditions that might cause **secondary hypertension**.

94. What is meant by the term **malignant hypertension**?

95. Identify **predisposing factors** for hypertension, indicating which ones are **modifiable**. Note that these parallel the risk factors for atherosclerosis and heart disease.

96. Describe the **pathophysiology and complications** of undiagnosed or uncontrolled hypertension.

97. Explain why hypertension is often referred to as **"the silent killer."**

98. Describe the **manifestations** of hypertension, distinguishing between early and later signs and symptoms.

99. Describe **lifestyle and behavioral changes** that are recommended in the treatment of hypertension. Explain the rationale for each modification.

100. What is the **greatest problem** in the treatment of hypertension?

ANITHYPERTENSIVE MEDICATIONS

101. Individuals with hypertension are often prescribed one or more antihypertensive medications, as well as other medications. Complete the following chart comparing and contrasting the most commonly prescribed types of **antihypertensive agents**:

Type of Antihypertensive	Mechanism of Action and Effects	Adverse Effects	Examples
Diuretics			
ACE inhibitors			
Calcium channel blockers			
β-adrenergic blockers			

102. Identify **adverse effects** that are common to **all** antihypertensive medications.

103. List other medications that might be prescribed, and state the rationale for each.

PERIPHERAL VASCULAR DISEASE (PVD)

104. Describe the **general manifestations** of peripheral vascular disease.

105. Outline the **therapeutic interventions** used in the treatment of peripheral vascular disease.

106. Complete the following chart comparing and contrasting **Buerger's disease and Raynaud's disease**:

	Buerger's Disease	Raynaud's Disease
High-risk groups		
Etiology		
Vessels involved		
Pathophysiology		
Manifestations		

107. Define **aneurysm**.

108. Identify the **causes** of aneurysms.

109. Describe the **complications** of aneurysms.

110. Identify factors that contribute to the **development of varicose veins**.

111. Describe the **manifestations** of varicosities.

112. Differentiate between **thrombophlebitis** and **phlebothrombosis**.

113. Identify three factors that contribute to the **development of thrombophlebitis**.

114. Outline measures that could **decrease** the risk of developing thrombophlebitis.

115. What is a **pulmonary embolus**? Where did the blood clot probably originate?

SHOCK

116. Define **shock**.

117. Outline the **compensatory mechanisms** that are recruited as the blood pressure decreases.

118. Describe the **general manifestations** of shock, including the cause of each.

119. Identify the **potential complications** of shock, and explain why each one occurs.

120. Outline general measures used in the **treatment** of shock.

121. Complete the following chart comparing and contrasting the **different types of shock**:

Type of Shock	Etiology	Specific Manifestations	Specific Treatment
Hypovolemic or hemorrhagic			
Cardiogenic			
Anaphylactic			
Septic			
Neurogenic (syncope)			

CONSOLIDATION

122. Identify the cardiovascular condition or conditions in which the following manifestations would be present:

i. ascites:

ii. positive Homan's sign:

iii. ECG changes:

iv. positive blood cultures:

v. claudication:

vi. hemoptysis:

vii. heart murmur:

viii. elevated cardiac enzymes:

ix. subcutaneous nodules:

x. pulmonary edema:

123. Identify the use or uses of the following drugs:

i. calcium channel blockers:

ii. nitroglycerine:

iii. penicillin:

iv. β-adrenergic blockers:

v. digoxin:

vi. diuretics:

vii. antiarrhythmics:

viii. ACE inhibitors:

19 Respiratory Disorders

1. Describe the common **complications of viral infections** of the respiratory tract.

2. Complete the following chart comparing and contrasting common childhood respiratory infections:

	Croup (Laryngotracheobronchitis)	Epiglottitis	Bronchiolitis
Usual age			
Cause			
Onset			
Pathology			
Significant manifestations			
Treatment			

3. Complete the following chart comparing and contrasting selected types of **pneumonia**:

	Lobar Pneumonia	Bronchial Pneumonia	Interstitial Pneumonia
Causative agent			
Onset			
Distribution within lungs			
Pathophysiology			
Manifestations			
Treatment			

4. Briefly describe *Pneumocystis carinii* **pneumonia (PCP)**. Identify individuals who are at high risk of contracting this type of pneumonia.

5. Name the microbial agent responsible for **SARS**, and identify its mode of transmission.

6. Outline the **pathophysiology** of SARS.

7. Describe the **manifestations** of SARS, including its effects on both blood gases and acid base balance.

8. Identify the therapeutic interventions used in the treatment of SARS.

9. Discuss the difficulties involved in controlling the spread of an infection when the causative agent is unidentified.

TUBERCULOSIS

10. Describe the characteristics of *Mycobacterium tuberculosis*.

11. Explain why it is difficult for host defensive cells to eradicate TB bacilli.

12. Identify individuals who are at **high risk** of contracting tuberculosis.

13. Describe the **pathophysiology** of tuberculosis, distinguishing between **primary** and **secondary infection**.

14. Describe the **lesion** that is **pathognomonic** for TB.

15. Outline the **manifestations** of tuberculosis, distinguishing between those that occur with primary infection and those that develop with secondary infection or re-infection.

16. Briefly describe **miliary tuberculosis**.

17. How is a diagnosis of active (i.e., infectious) tuberculosis **confirmed**?

18. What is a **Mantoux test**? What does a positive Mantoux indicate?

19. List **medications** used in the treatment of tuberculosis. Why is it necessary to take several different medications? What is the usual duration of drug therapy?

20. When will an individual who is taking TB medications become noncontagious? Explain why the drugs are prescribed for a longer period of time.

21. Individuals who are considered to be at high risk of contracting TB are routinely prescribed **TB prophylaxis**. Identify individuals who would be candidates for TB prophylaxis.

22. Identify the **medication** that is used for TB prophylaxis and the usual duration of treatment.

23. Describe measures that a **health care professional** should take to protect himself or herself against TB.

24. A patient/client states that his TB skin test has recently changed. What additional information should be obtained from this individual?

25. An individual states that he had TB a number of years ago. What additional information should be obtained from this patient/client?

CYSTIC FIBROSIS

26. What **type of disorder** is cystic fibrosis (CF)?

27. A baby is diagnosed with cystic fibrosis. Neither parent has this disorder. What are the genotypes of the parents? What is the probability that any of the baby's siblings will also have this disorder?

28. If an individual with cystic fibrosis had a child with an individual who was a carrier of CF, what is the probability that the child will have CF? What is the probability that he will be a carrier of CF?

29. Describe the **pathophysiology** of cystic fibrosis in detail.

30. Outline the **manifestations** of cystic fibrosis.

31. Identify tools used in the **diagnosis** of cystic fibrosis.

32. Outline the **therapeutic interventions** used in the treatment of cystic fibrosis.

33. What is the **life expectancy** of an individual with CF? What is the usual **cause of death**?

LUNG CANCER

34. Explain why the lungs are a frequent site of metastatic tumors.

35. List the **risk factors** for bronchogenic cancer.

36. Describe the **effects** of lung cancer.

37. Describe the **manifestations** of lung cancer.

38. List **therapeutic interventions** used in the treatment of lung cancer.

ASPIRATION

39. Define **aspiration**.

40. Identify individuals who are at **high risk** to aspirate something.

41. Describe the effects of aspiration.

42. Identify common **manifestations** of aspiration.

43. Describe the **Heimlich maneuver**.

ASTHMA

44. Define asthma.

45. Distinguish between **extrinsic and intrinsic asthma**.

46. Identify factors that commonly **precipitate** an asthmatic attack.

47. Describe the **pathophysiology** of an asthmatic attack, identifying the three factors that interfere with normal ventilation.

48. Outline the **potential complications** of poorly controlled asthma.

49. Describe the progression of an **asthmatic attack**.

50. Identify **nonpharmacological measures** used in the treatment of asthma.

51. Four types of **medications** are used in the control and treatment of asthma. Complete the following chart comparing and contrasting these drugs:

Drug Group	Action and Effects	Adverse Effects	Example and Route
Bronchodilators			
Corticosteroids			
Histamine release inhibitors			
Leukotriene receptor antagonists			

52. Identify which drug group can be used during as **acute asthmatic attack**. Why are the other three types ineffective in this situation?

53. Identify which type of medication has minimal adverse effects, is useful in preventing exercise-induced asthma, and is considered the safest for children with asthma?

54. An individual doesn't respond to his bronchodilator, and his asthma attack persists (i.e., status asthmaticus). What type of medication could be used at the hospital to relieve his symptoms?

55. An individual states he has asthma. What **additional information** should be obtained about his condition?

CHRONIC OBSTRUCTIVE PULMONARY DISEASE (COPD)

56. What is the **leading causative factor** for both emphysema and chronic bronchitis? Identify other **contributing factors** in the development of chronic obstructive pulmonary disease.

57. Explain why **polycythemia** may develop in both advanced emphysema and chronic bronchitis.

58. Identify the underlying **pathology** involved in **emphysema**.

59. Loss of alveolar walls characteristically occurs with emphysema. Explain the consequences of this change.

60. Explain why individuals with emphysema are sometimes referred to as **"pink puffers."**

61. Outline the **complications** that develop with the progression of emphysema.

62. What impact does increased residual volume have on blood gases in advanced emphysema? How could this affect blood pH?

63. Explain how respiratory control mechanisms change as emphysema progresses.

64. What is meant by the term **"barrel chest"**? Explain why this condition develops in individuals with emphysema.

65. Outline the **therapeutic interventions** used in the treatment of emphysema.

66. Describe the **pathophysiology of chronic bronchitis**.

67. Identify the **most significant symptom** of chronic bronchitis.

68. Explain why individuals with chronic bronchitis are sometimes referred to as **"blue bloaters"**?

69. Describe the **therapeutic interventions** employed in the treatment of chronic bronchitis.

70. Complete the following chart comparing and contrasting selected chronic obstructive lung disorders:

	Asthma	Emphysema	Chronic Bronchitis
Etiology and predisposing factor			
Location			
Pathophysiology			
Manifestations			
Complications			
Therapeutic interventions			

PULMONARY EDEMA

71. Identify the **causes** of pulmonary edema.

72. Describe the **pathophysiology** of pulmonary edema.

73. Describe the **manifestations** of pulmonary edema.

74. Explain why the sputum of an individual with pulmonary edema might be frothy and possibly pink in color.

75. Explain why an individual with mild pulmonary edema will experience dyspnea when he is placed in a supine position (e.g., for dental treatment). What is the term used to describe this condition?

76. Outline the treatment of pulmonary edema, including medications that might be used.

PULMONARY EMBOLUS

77. **Define** pulmonary embolus.

78. Where do most pulmonary emboli **originate**? Identify other **potential sources** of pulmonary emboli.

79. Identify individuals who are at **high risk** for developing pulmonary emboli.

80. Describe the **pathophysiology** of a pulmonary embolus.

81. Identify the **manifestations** of a pulmonary embolus.

82. What drugs may be used to **treat** pulmonary emboli?

EXPANSIVE DISORDERS

83. Explain the differences between **atelectasis** and **bronchiectasis**, including the etiologies and manifestations.

84. Explain the differences between a **pleural effusion** and **pneumothorax**, including etiologies and manifestations.

85. Explain what is meant by a **flail chest injury**?

86. Identify causes of **acute respiratory failure**.

87. Complete the following chart comparing and contrasting infant respiratory distress syndrome and adult respiratory distress syndrome:

	Infant Respiratory Distress Syndrome	Adult Respiratory Distress Syndrome
Etiology		
Pathophysiology		
Manifestations		
Treatment		

88. Match each of the following terms with the correct definition:

a) air in the pleural cavity

b) abnormal widening of the bronchi

c) excessive fluid in pleural cavity

d) chronic disorders resulting from continued exposure to irritating particles

e) fungal infection of the lungs

f) collapse of a portion of the lung

i) **pleural effusion** _____

ii) **atelectasis** _____

iii) **pneumothorax** _____

iv) **bronchiectasis** _____

v) **histoplasmosis** _____

vi) **pneumoconioses** _____

89. For each of the following characteristics or definitions, identify the appropriate respiratory disorder or disorders in which they occur:

    i. characterized by episodic bronchospasm:

    ii. causes orthopnea:

    iii. sputum often frothy and pink or blood-tinged:

    iv. loss of alveolar walls and lung elasticity:

    v. caused by an acid-fast bacillus:

    vi. acute manifestations usually relieved by adrenergic agonists:

    vii. occurs most commonly in immunosuppressed individuals:

    viii. deficit of pancreatic digestive enzymes:

    ix. collapse of a lung or portion of a lung:

    x. characterized by a constant productive cough:

    xi. a potential complication of thrombophlebitis in leg veins:

    xii. inadequate production of surfactant:

    xiii. results from rib fractures:

    xiv. defect in chloride ion transport in cell membranes:

    xv. causes malabsorption of nutrients:

    xvi. may cause cavitation within lungs:

xvii. abnormal dilation of the bronchi:

xviii. accumulation of fluid in the pleural cavity:

xix. characterized by caseation necrosis:

xx. treated with leukotriene receptor antagonists:

20 Digestive System Disorders

1. Match the following terms with the correct definition:

   a) drug used to decrease nausea and vomiting

   b) formation of gallstones

   c) greasy, loose stools

   d) loss of appetite

   e) opportunistic oral fungal infection

   f) outpouching of the mucosa in colon

   g) tarry stools caused by bleeding

   h) difficulty swallowing

   i) inflammation of tissue surrounding the teeth

   j) retention of feces

   k) vomit containing blood

   i) steatorrhea _____

   ii) melena _____

   iii) dysphagia _____

   iv) antiemetic _____

   v) anorexia _____

   vi) hematemesis _____

   vii) impaction _____

   viii) candidiasis _____

   ix) gingivitis _____

   viii) cholelithiasis _____

   xi) diverticulum _____

2. Identify six causes of vomiting, and state an example of each.

3. Outlines measures that are used to decrease vomiting.

4. Identify seven causes of constipation.

5. What dietary modifications could help relieve chronic constipation?

6. Identify the causes of **dysphagia**.

7. Describe a **hiatal hernia**.

8. Describe the **manifestations** of a hiatal hernia.

9. Outline the **therapeutic interventions** used in the treatment of hiatal hernia.

10. What is **GERD**? Identify the **etiology** of GERD.

11. What types of medications are used in the treatment of GERD?

12. Distinguish between acute gastritis and acute gastroenteritis.

13. Differentiate between acute gastritis and chronic gastritis in relation to etiology and manifestations.

14. Complete the following chart comparing and contrasting selected types of **food poisoning**:

Pathogen	Source	Incubation	Manifestations
Staphylococcus aureus			
Escherichia coli (*E. coli,* "traveler's diarrhea," or "hamburger disease")			
Salmonella			
Clostridium botulinum			

15. State the **locations** where ulcers occur.

16. Identify **factors** that contribute to the development of peptic ulcers.

17. Describe the **pathophysiology** of peptic ulcers.

18. Outline the **potential complications** that may occur with peptic ulcers.

19. Describe the **manifestations** of peptic ulcers.

20. Identify the **therapeutic interventions** used in the treatment of ulcers.

CANCER

21. Complete the following chart comparing and contrasting **cancer** of the gastrointestinal tract and accessory organ:

	Etiology	Pathophysiology	Manifestations and Complications	Treatment
Esophagus				
Stomach				
Liver				
Pancreas				
Colorectal				

GALLBLADDER DISEASE

22. Identify individuals who are considered **high risk** for developing **gallstones**.

23. Describe the **manifestations of gallstones**.

LIVER DISEASE

24. State the three classes of disorders that may cause **jaundice**, and state several examples of each.

25. Identify **causes** of **nonviral hepatitis**.

26. Complete the following chart comparing and contrasting the most common types of **viral hepatitis**:

	Hepatitis A	Hepatitis B	Hepatitis C
Causative agent			
Transmission			
High-risk groups			
Age			
Incubation period			
Severity of symptoms			
Duration of manifestations			
Carrier state			
Complications			

	Hepatitis A, cont'd	Hepatitis B, cont'd	Hepatitis C, cont'd
Serological markers			
Medications			
Immunoglobulin			
Vaccine			

27. Explain what is meant by the **"fecal-oral"** route of transmission. State several examples of how infections can be spread this way.

28. **Hepatitis D** occurs only in individuals who also have hepatitis B. Explain why.

29. How can **hepatitis D** infection be detected if the person also has hepatitis B?

30. How is **hepatitis E** contracted?

31. The manifestations of all types of hepatitis are remarkably similar. What varies is the onset, severity, and duration of symptoms. Describe the **general manifestations** of hepatitis.

32. A client/patient states that he has had hepatitis. Identify **additional information** that should be obtained from this individual.

33. Define **cirrhosis**.

34. Identify **causes of cirrhosis**.

35. Describe the **pathophysiology** of cirrhosis.

36. Identify the **liver functions** that are lost or impaired with cirrhosis.

37. Describe the **manifestations** that result as a consequence of the losses identified in the previous question.

38. Explain what is meant by **portal hypertension** and how it develops.

39. Describe the **complications** that develop as a consequence of portal hypertension.

40. Outline the **therapeutic interventions** used in the treatment of cirrhosis.

PANCREATITIS

41. Identify the **causes** of acute pancreatitis.

42. Describe the **pathophysiology** of acute pancreatitis.

43. Identify the **manifestations** of pancreatitis.

44. Outline the **treatment** of pancreatitis.

INTESTINAL DISORDERS

45. What is **celiac disease**?

46. Briefly describe the **pathophysiology** of celiac disease.

47. What are the characteristic manifestations of malabsorption syndromes?

48. Outline the **treatment** of celiac disease.

49. Describe the **pathophysiology** of appendicitis.

50. Outline the **manifestations** of acute appendicitis.

51. Explain what is meant by **chronic inflammatory bowel disease**.

52. Complete the following chart comparing and contrasting Crohn's disease and ulcerative colitis:

	Crohn's Disease	Ulcerative Colitis
Individuals at high risk		
Etiology		
Location of lesions		
Characteristics of lesions		
Complications		
Manifestations		

53. Describe the **therapeutic interventions** used in the treatment of inflammatory bowel disease.

54. Briefly describe the **pathophysiology** and **complications** of diverticulitis.

55. List the **warning signs** of **colorectal cancer**.

56. State **causes** of **intestinal obstruction**.

57. Outline the **pathophysiology and complications** of intestinal obstruction.

58. Describe the **manifestations** of intestinal obstruction.

59. Define **peritonitis**.

60. Identify the **causes** of peritonitis.

61. Outline the **pathophysiology and complications** of peritonitis.

62. Describe the **manifestations** of peritonitis.

63. Identify **therapeutic interventions** used in the treatment of peritonitis.

CONSOLIDATION

64. Identify the classification of the following medications, and state at least one condition for which each would be prescribed:

    i. prednisone:

    ii. dimenhydrinate:

    iii. clarithromycin:

    iv. ranitidine:

    v. loperamide:

    vi. psyllium:

    vii. sucralfate:

21 Urinary System Disorders

1. Explain the difference between **hemodialysis** and **peritoneal dialysis**.

2. Identify **potential complications of hemodialysis**.

3. Explain why individuals receiving hemodialysis are at an **increased risk** of developing HIV and hepatitis B and C.

4. Individuals who require dialysis are usually required to take **prophylactic antibiotics** before dental treatment or other invasive procedures. Explain why the administration of antibiotics is necessary.

5. Identify factors that **predispose** an individual to the development of a **urinary tract infection**. Explain why females are more prone to urinary tract infections than men.

6. Distinguish between the **manifestations** of **cystitis** and **pyelonephritis**.

7. Describe the **pathophysiology** of **glomerulonephritis**.

8. Outline the **manifestations** of glomerulonephritis.

9. Identify tests use to **diagnose** glomerulonephritis.

10. Describe the **pathophysiology** of **nephrotic syndrome**.

11. Identify the **most significant manifestation** of nephrotic syndrome, and outline the potental consequences.

12. List the **medications** used in the treatment of nephrotic syndrome.

13. Identify **causative factors** in the development of **renal calculi**.

14. Individuals with renal calculi are routinely instructed to strain their urine. Explain the rationale for this procedure.

15. Identify the characteristic **manifestations** of renal calculi.

16. Define **hydronephrosis**.

17. Identify **causes** of hydronephrosis.

18. Define **nephrosclerosis**.

19. List the **causes** of nephrosclerosis.

RENAL FAILURE

20. Identify **causes** of **acute renal failure**.

21. Outline the **treatment** of acute renal failure.

22. Identify **causes** of **chronic renal failure**.

23. Distinguish between **renal insufficiency** and **end-stage renal failure**.

24. Describe the **manifestations** of end-stage renal failure under the following headings:

    i. fluid and electrolyte balance:

    ii. cardiovascular system:

    iii. central nervous system:

    iv. musculoskeletal system:

    v. endocrine system:

    vi. skin and mucosa:

25. Explain why each of the following manifestations occurs in end-stage renal failure:

     i. metabolic acidosis:

     ii. hyperkalemia:

     iii. hypocalcemia:

     iv. increased BUN and serum creatinine:

     v. anemia:

     vi. delayed clotting:

     vii. edema:

     viii. increased blood pressure:

     ix. cardiac arrhythmias:

     x. congestive heart failure:

     xi. pulmonary edema:

     xii. lethargy, confusion:

     xiii. muscle weakness:

     xiv. bone tenderness:

     xv. amenorrhea:

     xvi. severe pruritus:

     xvii. ammonia odor on breath:

     xviii. hypoplasia of tooth enamel:

26. Individuals with renal failure have an increased chance of having an exaggerated or prolonged response to many medications. Explain why.

27. Complete the following crossword puzzle:

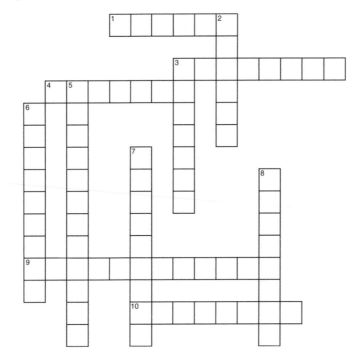

ACROSS
1. presence of pus in the urine
3. medication that promotes urination
4. sudden, extreme urge to void
9. inability to control urination
10. scanty urine output

DOWN
2. no urine output
3. painful urination
5. kidney stones
6. blood in the urine
7. inability to empty bladder
8. presence of nitrogenous wastes in blood

22 Acute Neurologic Disorders

1. Identify conditions in which **increased intracranial pressure** may develop.

2. Describe the **consequences** of increased intracranial pressure.

3. Identify the **manifestations** of increased intracranial pressure, explaining why each one occurs.

TUMORS

4. Manifestations of brain tumors, whether they originate in the brain or are metastatic tumors, are primarily caused by their space-occupying effect and the replacement of normal tissue by tumor cells. Summarize the potential **generalized manifestations** of brain tumors (i.e., nonfocal).

TIAs AND CVAs

5. Define **transient ischemic attack (TIA)**.

6. Describe the **manifestations** of a TIA.

7. Explain the **significance** of TIAs.

8. Differentiate between a TIA and a cerebrovascular accident (CVA).

9. Identify individuals who are considered to be at **high risk** for experiencing a CVA or stroke.

10. Describe the **warning signs** of a stroke. Notice that they are the same as the manifestations of a transient ischemic attack.

11. Identify the three common **categories of cerebrovascular accident** or stroke, indicating which one occurs most commonly.

12. Describe the **pathophysiology** of a cerebrovascular accident.

13. Complete the following chart comparing and contrasting the three most common types of cerebrovascular accidents:

	Thrombus CVA	Embolus CVA	Hemorrhage CVA
Predisposing factors			
Onset			
Effects			
Immediate treatment			
Prognosis			

14. Identify the possible origins of **cerebral emboli**.

15. Explain why the **prognosis** for a hemorrhagic type stroke is worse than for other types.

16. Describe the possible **manifestations** of a CVA under the following headings:

    i. motor deficits:

    ii. sensory deficits:

    iii. speech deficits:

    iv. cognitive and emotional manifestations:

17. Describe the **therapeutic interventions** used in the long term treatment of an individual who has experienced a CVA, including medications.

18. An individual suffers a massive thrombus-type CVA involving his left frontal and parietal lobes. Describe the manifestations that he would probably experience.

ANEURYSMS

19. Define **aneurysm**.

20. Identify the most common factor that precipitates **rupture** of an aneurysm.

21. Describe **manifestations** of both an enlarging and a ruptured aneurysm.

INFECTIONS

22. Complete the following chart comparing and contrasting **meningitis and encephalitis**:

	Meningitis	Encephalitis
Causative agents		
Predisposing factors		
Pathophysiology		
Manifestations		
Treatment		

23. Identify the location of the following **head injuries**:

    i. basilar fracture:

    ii. epidural hematoma:

    iii. subdural hematoma:

    iv. subarachnoid hematoma:

    v. intracranial hematoma:

24. Describe the **consequences and potential complications** of a head injury.

25. Describe the **general manifestations** of head injuries.

26. Identify therapeutic interventions employed in the **treatment** of a head injury.

27. Identify the common **causes** of **spinal cord injuries**.

28. Outline the **consequences and potential complications** of a spinal cord injury.

29. Describe the potential **manifestations** of a spinal cord injury.

30. Identify the **therapeutic interventions** used in treatment of spinal cord injuries.

31. Complete the following crossword puzzle:

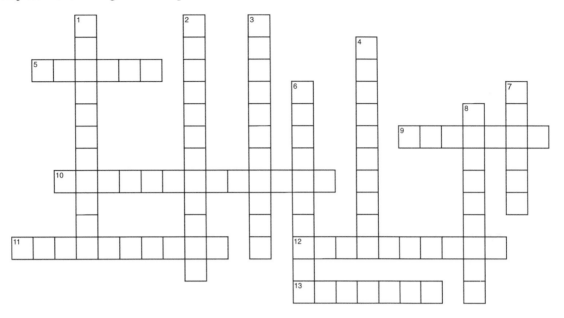

ACROSS
  5. drooping eyelid
  9. inability to recognize everyday objects
10. opposite side
11. difficulty pronouncing words
12. paralysis of lower half of body
13. inability to express or comprehend speech

DOWN
  1. increased sensitivity to light
  2. paralysis of all four limbs
  3. same side
  4. paralysis of one side of body
  6. loss of vision from the medial side of one eye and the lateral side of the other eye
  7. brain tumor originating in neuroglial cells
  8. bruising of the brain

23 Chronic Neurologic Disorders

HYDROCEPHALUS

1. Define **hydrocephalus**.

2. State the **causes** of hydrocephalus.

3. Outline the **pathophysiology** of hydrocephalus.

4. Distinguish between **noncommunicating** (obstructive) and **communicating** hydrocephalus.

5. Describe the **manifestations** of hydrocephalus.

6. What is the **treatment** for hydrocephalus?

SPINA BIFIDA

7. Identify the **basic defect** involved in spina bifida.

8. Describe the three **types** of spina bifida.

9. How is spina bifida **diagnosed** prenatally?

10. List the possible **causes** of spina bifida.

11. Describe the **manifestations** of spina bifida.

12. Outline the **treatment** of spina bifida.

CEREBRAL PALSY

13. List the **causes** of cerebral palsy.

14. Describe the **pathophysiology** of cerebral palsy.

15. Describe the three major classifications of **motor disabilities** that occur with cerebral palsy.

16. Identify other possible **manifestations** of cerebral palsy.

17. Outline the **treatment** of cerebral palsy.

SEIZURE DISORDERS

18. Define **seizure**.

19. Describe the **pathophysiology** of a seizure disorder.

20. Distinguish between **primary and secondary (acquired) seizures**.

21. List **causes** of acquired seizures.

22. Differentiate between a **generalized seizure** and a **partial seizure**.

23. Describe an **absence**, or **petit mal, seizure**. What is the usual **duration** of this type of seizure?

24. What is meant by **prodromal signs**?

25. What is an **aura**? Give several examples of typical auras. What is the significance of an aura?

26. Identify factors that might **precipitate a seizure** in an individual who suffers from epilepsy.

27. Describe a **tonic clonic seizure**. What is the typical **duration** of this type of seizure?

28. What are the **potential complications** of a seizure?

29. Outline the **emergency treatment** of a seizure.

30. When is it necessary to seek **medical assistance**?

31. Differentiate between a **simple partial** and a **complex partial seizure**.

32. Identify two types of **medications** prescribed to prevent seizures.

33. Describe the **adverse effects** of these drugs.

34. What is **status epilepticus**? What drugs are used to treat this condition?

35. An individual states that he suffers from epilepsy. What **additional information** should you obtain before initiating treatment?

36. What measures should be taken to decrease the possibility of precipitating a seizure?

MULTIPLE SCLEROSIS (MS)

37. What is the **etiology** of multiple sclerosis (MS)?

38. Identify individuals who are at **high risk** for developing multiple sclerosis.

39. Describe the **pathological changes** that occur with multiple sclerosis. What is a **plaque**?

40. What **type of neurons** are affected by multiple sclerosis?

41. How is MS **diagnosed**?

42. Describe the **manifestations** of multiple sclerosis, distinguishing between early and late symptoms.

43. Outline the **therapeutic interventions** used in the treatment of MS.

44. Explain the rationale for the use of corticosteroids and interferon in the treatment of MS.

45. State the underlying **pathological change** that occurs in Parkinson's disease. Describe the consequences of this change.

46. Describe the **manifestations** of Parkinson's, distinguishing between early and later symptoms.

47. What drug group may cause **pseudoparkinsonism**?

48. List drug groups that are used in the **treatment** of Parkinson's disease.

ALS, MYASTHENIA GRAVIS, HUNTINGTON'S DISEASE

49. Amyotrophic lateral sclerosis, myasthenia gravis, and Huntington's disease are all progressive neurological disorders that cause motor deficits. Complete the following chart comparing and contrasting these three conditions:

	Amyotrophic Lateral Sclerosis	Myasthenia Gravis	Huntington's Disease
Etiology			
Pathophysiology			
Manifestations			
Treatment			
Prognosis			

50. State several **causes** of dementia.

51. Outline the typical changes that occur in the brains of individuals with **Alzheimer's disease**.

52. List the **causes** of **Alzheimer's disease**.

53. Identify the **manifestations** of Alzheimer's disease.

MENTAL ILLNESS

54. Summarize the types of **behavior** exhibited by individuals with **schizophrenia**.

55. Describe the **adverse effects** of **antipsychotic medications**.

56. Identify **types of antidepressant drugs**, and state an example of each.

HERNIATED DISK

57. Describe the herniation of an intervertebral disk.

58. What is the most serious **complication** of a herniated disk?

59. Identify the **most common site** of a herniated disk, and describe the resulting **manifestations**.

60. Outline the **treatment** of a herniated lumbar disk.

CONSOLIDATION

61. A client has a history of **cognitive impairment**. What **additional information** should you try to obtain?

62. Identify how treatment should be modified for an individual with a history of cognitive impairment.

63. For each of the following pathological findings/characteristics, identify the condition or conditions in which they occur:

    i. loss of myelin in the CNS:

    ii. impairment of receptors at neuromuscular junctions:

    iii. deterioration of basal ganglia:

    iv. development of neurofibrillary tangles:

    v. decreased dopamine synthesis:

    vi. depletion of GABA:

    vii. degeneration of both upper and lower motor neurons:

    viii. an autosomal dominant disorder:

    ix. an autoimmune disorder:

    x. characterized by rigidity and difficulty initiating movements:

    xi. development of plaques in the brain:

    xii. decreased levels of Ach in the CNS:

    xiii. treated with levodopa:

    xiv. treated with donepezil:

    xv. caused by infection by a prion:

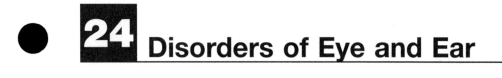

24 Disorders of Eye and Ear

EYE

1. State the **basic pathology** involved in glaucoma.

2. Differentiate between **narrow-angle** and **wide-angle** glaucoma.

3. Identify individuals who are at **increased risk** of developing glaucoma.

4. List the **manifestations** of glaucoma.

5. Outline the therapeutic interventions used in the **treatment** of glaucoma.

6. Complete the following chart comparing and contrasting common ocular problems:

	Cataract	Macular Degeneration	Detached Retina
Etiology			
Pathology			
Effect on vision			
Treatment			

7. For each of the following pathological findings/characteristics, identify the condition(s) in which they occur:

    i. characterized by clouding of the ocular lens:

    ii. characterized by degeneration of the fovea centralis:

    iii. treated with cholinergic eye drops:

    iv. characterized by loss of central vision:

    v. appearances of "halos" around lights:

    vi. increased intraocular pressure:

EAR

8. Differentiate between conduction deafness and sensorineural deafness, and state several examples of each type.

9. Briefly outline the pathophysiology of Meniere's disease.

10. Describe the manifestations of Meniere's disease.

11. Identify individuals who are at high risk for developing the following conditions:

    i. otitis media:

    ii. otitis externa:

25 Endocrine Disorders

DIABETES MELLITUS

1. List the **predisposing factors** for developing diabetes mellitus.

2. Describe the **etiology** of diabetes mellitus, comparing **type I** and **type II**.

3. Describe in detail the **pathophysiology** of diabetes mellitus.

4. Explain why **ketoacidosis** develops in untreated or uncontrolled diabetes mellitus.

5. Identify the **warning signs** of diabetes mellitus, explaining the pathological basis for each manifestation.

6. How is a **diagnosis** of diabetes mellitus established?

7. Outline the **dietary modifications** that are required in the successful treatment of diabetes mellitus.

8. How do **oral hypoglycemic or antidiabetic agents** lower blood sugar?

9. Explain why individuals with type I diabetes mellitus cannot be treated with oral hypogolycemics.

10. List the **adverse effects** of oral antidiabetic agents.

11. What are the differences among the various forms of **insulin**?

12. How is insulin administered?

13. Identify factors that could precipitate a **hypoglycemic or insulin reaction**.

14. Identify measures that could minimize the chances of a diabetic individual experiencing a hypoglycemic reaction.

15. Distinguish between **microangiopathy and macroangiopathy**, including the consequences of each.

16. Explain what is meant by **diabetic neuropathy**. Identify the cause and complications of diabetic neuropathy.

17. Explain why individuals with diabetes are considered to be at high risk for developing **infections**.

18. Identify the **types of infections** that commonly occur in individuals with poorly regulated diabetes mellitus.

19. Explain why there may be **delayed healing** in an individual with diabetes mellitus.

20. What is **gestational diabetes**?

21. A client states that she has diabetes mellitus. What additional information should you obtain from her?

22. Complete the following chart comparing and contrasting the two **acute complications** that may occur in an individual who has diabetes:

	Hypoglycemic Shock	Ketoacidosis
Other names		
Cause		
Precipitating factors		
Speed of onset		
Manifestations		

	Hypoglycemic Shock, cont'd	Ketoacidosis, cont'd
Emergency treatment		
Speed of response to emergency treatment		
Prevention		

23. Complete the following chart comparing and contrasting type I and type II diabetes mellitus:

	Type I (IDDM)	Type II (NIDDM)
Percentage of individuals with DM		
Age at onset		
Speed of onset of symptoms		
Family history		
Body build		

(cont'd)

	Type I (IDDM), cont'd	Type II (NIDDM), cont'd
Presence of autoantibodies		
Insulin receptor defects		
Severity of manifestations		
Stability (i.e., maintenance of normal blood glucose)		
Frequency of complications		
Occurrence of ketoacidosis		
Frequency of hypoglycemia		
Treatment with insulin		
Treatment with oral hypoglycemics		

PARATHYROID DISORDERS

24. Identify the **consequences** of **hypoparathyroidism**.

25. Identify the **consequences** of **hyperparathyroidism**.

ACROMEGALY

26. State the **etiology** of acromegaly.

27. Outline the **manifestations and complications** of acromegaly.

THYROID DISORDERS

28. What is a **goiter**? Identify the **etiology** of a goiter.

29. Complete the following chart comparing and contrasting **hyperthyroidism** and **hypothyroidism**:

	Hyperthyroidism	Hypothyroidism
Forms		
Etiology		
Serum T_3 and T_4 levels		
Metabolic rate		
Nervous system effects		
Cardiovascular effects		
Respiratory effects		
Skeletal effects		
Muscular effects		

(cont'd)

	Hyperthyroidism, cont'd	Hypothyroidism, cont'd
Skin and hair		
Temperature tolerance		
Eyes		
Body weight		
Presence of goiter		
Treatment		

ADRENAL DISORDERS

30. Complete the following chart comparing and contrasting **Cushing's syndrome** and **Addison's disease**:

	Cushing's Syndrome	Addison's Disease
Etiology		
Physical appearance		
Fluid and electrolytes		
Blood pressure		
Blood sugar		
Musculoskeletal effects		

	Cushing's Syndrome, cont'd	Addison's Disease, cont'd
Inflammatory response		
Immune response		
Response to stress		
Treatment		

31. Individuals with Cushing's syndrome may be prescribed prophylactic antibacterial drugs before invasive procedures such as dental surgery. Explain the rationale for this.

CONSOLIDATION

32. For each of the following disorders, identify the etiology (i.e., hyposecretion or hypersecretion of a specific hormone):

   i. Graves' disease:

   ii. gigantism:

   iii. myxedema:

   iv. diabetes insipidus:

   v. acromegaly:

   vi. Cushing's syndrome:

   vii. dwarfism:

   viii. diabetes mellitus:

ix. Addison's disease:

x. cretinism:

33. For each of the following characteristics, identify the endocrine disorder or disorders in which they occur:

    i. hyperglycemia:

    ii. increased basal metabolic rate:

    iii. increased susceptibility to infection:

    iv. intolerance to cold:

    v. development of osteoporosis or decreased bone density:

    vi. mental retardation:

    vii. predisposition to renal calculi:

    viii. hypotension:

    ix. impaired physical growth:

    x. hyperpigmentation of the skin and oral mucosa:

    xi. an autoimmune disorder:

    xii. development of peripheral edema:

    xiii. development of exophthalmos:

    xiv. bradycardia:

    xv. delayed clotting:

    xvi. poor healing:

xvii. poor response to stress:

xviii. development or exacerbation of hypertension:

xix. weight loss:

xx. presence of a goiter:

xxi. enlarged hands and feet:

xxii. tachycardia and palpitations:

xxiii. hyponatremia:

xxiv. hypocalcemia:

Chapter 25 Endocrine Disorders

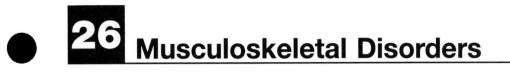

26 Musculoskeletal Disorders

1. Outline the **distinguishing characteristics** of the following types of fractures:

    i. compound:

    ii. comminuted:

    iii. compression:

    iv. greenstick:

    v. impacted:

    vi. oblique:

    vii. pathological:

    viii. spiral:

    ix. transverse:

    x. Colles':

2. Describe in detail the **healing of a closed transverse fracture**.

3. Identify the **potential complications** of fractures.

4. What is meant by **"reduction"** of a fracture? Differentiate between a closed reduction and an open reduction.

5. Explain the difference between a joint **dislocation and subluxation**.

6. Differentiate between a **sprain and an avulsion**.

7. List factors that **predispose** an individual to osteoporosis.

8. Identify **common sites** of osteoporosis.

9. Describe the **pathophysiology** of osteoporosis.

10. Outline the **treatment** of osteoporosis, including the rationale for each therapeutic intervention.

11. Complete the following chart comparing and contrasting **rickets, osteomalacia, and Paget's disease**:

	Rickets	Osteomalacia	Paget's Disease
Etiology			
Manifestations			
Treatment			

12. Identify a drug group that may cause osteomalacia with prolonged use.

13. Differentiate between an **osteosarcoma and a chondrosarcoma**.

MUSCULAR DYSTROPHY

14. Describe the underlying **pathology** involved in muscular dystrophy.

15. Complete the following chart comparing and contrasting the four types of **muscular dystrophy**:

	Duchenne's	Fascioscapulo-Humeral	Myotonic	Limb Girdle
Mode of inheritance				
Age of onset				
Muscle involvement				
Progression				

FIBROMYALGIA

16. Identify the **manifestations** of fibromyalgia.

ARTHRITIS

17. Explain why osteoarthritis is often referred to as **"wear-and-tear arthritis."**

18. Complete the following chart comparing and contrasting osteoarthritis and rheumatoid arthritis:

	Osteoarthritis	Rheumatoid Arthritis
Etiology		
Predisposing factors		
Joints involved		
Pathophysiology		
Manifestations		
Extra-articular manifestations		
Treatment		

19. Identify **drug types** that may be used in the treatment of rheumatoid arthritis.

20. Outline how **juvenile rheumatoid arthritis** differs from the adult form.

21. Identify the basic underlying problem with **gout**.

22. Outline how **gout** differs from other forms of arthritis.

23. Describe the **pathological changes** that occur in **ankylosing spondylitis**.

CONSOLIDATION

24. Identify the disease or diseases for which each of the following statements or characteristics is true:

    i. loss of articular cartilage:

    ii. development of tophi in soft tissue, bone, or both:

    iii. possible presence of an antibody against IgG in the serum:

    iv. classified as an autoimmune disease:

    v. presence of extraarticular (i.e., systemic) manifestations:

    vi. a sex-linked disorder:

    vii. may be treated with estrogen replacement therapy:

    viii. most commonly affects weight-bearing joints:

    ix. highest incidence in women between the ages of 20 and 50:

    x. characterized by synovitis and pannus formation:

    xi. treatment may involve intra-articular injections of glucocorticoids:

    xii. may result in the development of kyphosis:

    xiii. may be accompanied by ocular complications such as uveitis:

    xiv. affects joints in hands and feet:

    xv. characterized by elevated serum uric acid levels:

    xvi. development of ankylosis or joint fusion over time:

xvii. treated with NSAIDs:

xviii. immunosuppressants sometimes prescribed during exacerbations:

xix. characterized by the development of osteophytes:

xx. primary involvement occurs in the intervertebral joints:

xxi. characterized by compression fractures of the vertebral bodies:

xxii. crepitus often present:

xxiii. treated with bisphosphonates:

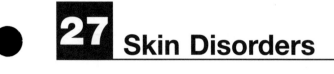

27 Skin Disorders

1. State the **etiology** for each of the following skin conditions. Be as specific as possible: If the cause is an infection, identify the causative organism. Also identify the treatment for each condition.

Condition	Etiology	Treatment
Scleroderma		
Kaposi's sarcoma		
Tinea		
Atopic dermatitis		
Pemphigus		
Herpes zoster		
Herpes simplex		
Verruca		
Urticaria		

(cont'd)

Condition, cont'd	Etiology, cont'd	Treatment, cont'd
Psoriasis		
Scabies		
Lichen planus		
Impetigo		
Cellulitis		
Necrotizing fasciitis		

2. Identify individuals who are at **high risk** for developing each of the following **malignancies**:

    i. squamous cell carcinoma:

    ii. malignant melanoma:

    iii. Kaposi's sarcoma:

3. Complete the following crossword puzzle:

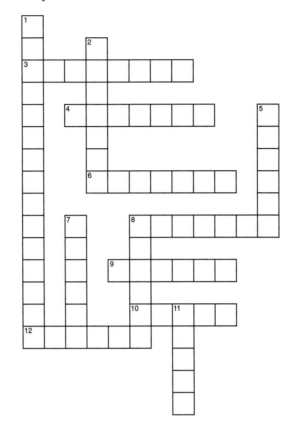

ACROSS
  3. mass of sebum, keratin, and debris blocking the opening of a hair follicle
  4. small, deep linear crack or tear in skin
  6. shallow, moist cavity in epidermis
  8. elevated, erythematous lesion, usually containing purulent exudates
  9. small, firm, elevated lesion
  10. cavity with loss of tissue from the epidermis and dermis, often weeping or bleeding
  12. palpable elevated lesion; varies in size

DOWN
  1. thick, dry, rough surface (leatherlike)
  2. elevated, thin-walled lesion containing clear fluid (blister)
  5. small, flat, circumscribed lesion of a different color than the normal skin
  7. raised, irregular, and increasing mass of collagen resulting from excessive scar tissue formation
  8. large, slightly elevated lesion with flat surface, often topped by scale
  11. dry, rough surface or dried exudates or blood

CONSOLIDATION

4. Identify the disease or diseases for which each of the following statements or characteristics is true:

  i. most commonly associated with HIV and AIDS:

ii. commonly known as hives:

iii. an autoimmune disorder that results in blister formation:

iv. associated with chicken pox:

v. caused by a mite:

vi. commonly known as coldsores:

vii. caused by human papillomavirus:

viii. superficial fungal infection:

ix. commonly known as eczema:

x. characterized by thickening of both the dermis and epidermis:

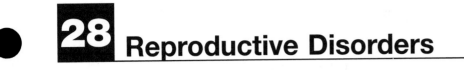

28 Reproductive Disorders

1. Identify causes of **infertility** in both males and females.

MALES

2. Define the following terms:

    i. **hypospadias**:

    ii. **epispadias**:

    iii. **cryptorchidism**:

    iv. **hydrocele**:

    v. **spermatocele**:

    vi. **varicocele**:

3. State factors that **predispose** a man to the development of **prostatitis**.

4. What is the most common **causative agent** in bacterial prostatitis?

5. Outline the **manifestations** of prostatitis.

6. Describe **benign prostatic hypertrophy**.

7. Explain how benign prostatic hypertrophy could lead to cystitis and kidney damage.

8. Identify the **manifestations** of benign prostatic hypertrophy.

9. What are the **risk factors** associated with the development of **prostatic cancer**?

10. What are the **warning or early signs** of **prostatic cancer**?

11. Prostatic cancer often metastasizes. Identify common **sites of metastases**.

12. What **screening tool** is useful in the early detection of prostatic cancer?

13. Why is surgical removal of the testes sometimes useful in the treatment of prostatic cancer?

14. List known **risk factors** for **testicular cancer**.

15. Describe the **manifestations** of testicular cancer.

16. Outline **therapeutic interventions** used in the treatment of testicular cancer.

FEMALE

17. Define the following terms:

   i. **anteflexion**:

   ii. **retroflexion**:

   iii. **cystocele**:

   iv. **rectocele**:

   v. **uterine prolapse**:

   vi. **dysmenorrhea**:

   vii. **amenorrhea**:

   viii. **dyspareunia**:

ENDOMETRIOSIS

18. What is **endometriosis**?

19. Describe the **pathophysiology** of endometriosis.

20. Identify the **chief complaint** with endometriosis.

21. Outline the **treatment** for endometriosis.

VAGINAL CANDIDIASIS

22. Identify **predisposing factors** for the development of **vaginal candidiasis**. Note that these are exactly the same factors that predispose an individual to oral candidiasis.

23. Outline the **manifestations** of vaginal candidiasis.

PELVIC INFLAMMATORY DISEASE (PID)

24. Define **pelvic inflammatory disease (PID)**.

25. Identify **predisposing factors** for the development of pelvic inflammatory disease.

26. Describe the **pathophysiology** of pelvic inflammatory disease.

27. Outline the **manifestations** of pelvic inflammatory disease.

28. Identify the potential complications of untreated pelvic inflammatory disease.

29. What is the **treatment** for pelvic inflammatory disease?

CERVICAL CANCER

30. Explain why the number of deaths from cervical cancer has declined. Why has the incidence of new cases not decreased?

31. Identify individuals who are considered at **high risk** for developing cervical cancer.

32. Describe the **progression** of undiagnosed or untreated cervical cancer.

33. List the **signs and symptoms** of cervical cancer.

34. Outline the **treatment** for cervical cancer.

ENDOMETRIAL CANCER

35. Identify individuals who are considered at **high risk** for developing endometrial cancer.

36. Describe the **progression** of undiagnosed or untreated endometrial cancer.

37. List the **manifestations** of endometrial cancer.

38. Outline the **treatment** of endometrial cancer.

BREAST CANCER

39. Identify the **risk factors** for breast cancer.

40. Outline the **development** of breast cancer, including **metastatic pattern**.

41. Identify the **manifestations** of breast cancer.

42. Outline the **therapeutic interventions** used in the treatment of breast cancer.

43. Discuss measures that can be used to detect **early signs** of breast cancer.

44. Complete the following chart comparing and contrasting different sexually transmitted diseases:

Infection	Causative Agent	Manifestations	Complications	Treatment
Chlamydia				
Gonorrhea				
Syphilis				
Genital herpes				
Genital warts				
Trichomoniasis				

Answer Key

CHAPTER 1

Introduction to Pathophysiology

1. (pp. 10-12)
   - i. hyperplasia
   - ii. hyperplasia
   - iii. atrophy
   - iv. hypertrophy
   - v. hypertrophy
   - vi. atrophy
   - vii. atrophy
   - viii. hyperplasia
   - ix. hypertrophy
   - x. atrophy
   - xi. metaplasia; dysplasia; neoplasia
   - xii. dysplasia
   - xiii. hypertrophy
   - xiv. hyperplasia
   - xv. atrophy
   - xvi. hyperplasia
   - xvii. hyperplasia
   - xviii. hypertrophy
   - xix. hyperplasia
   - xx. hypertrophy
2. (p. 11) dysplasia; it is the forerunner of neoplasia
3. (p. 12) failure of cells to differentiate or develop specialized features; term applied to grading malignant tumors
4. (p. 12)
   - i. ischemia
   - ii. physical agents, e.g., excessive temperature, radiation
   - iii. mechanical damage
   - iv. chemical toxins or foreign substances
   - v. pathogens
   - vi. abnormal metabolites
   - vii. nutritional deficits

   or

   - vii. fluid or electrolyte imbalances
5. answer to crossword puzzle (see below)
6. (See Fig. 1-2, p. 11)

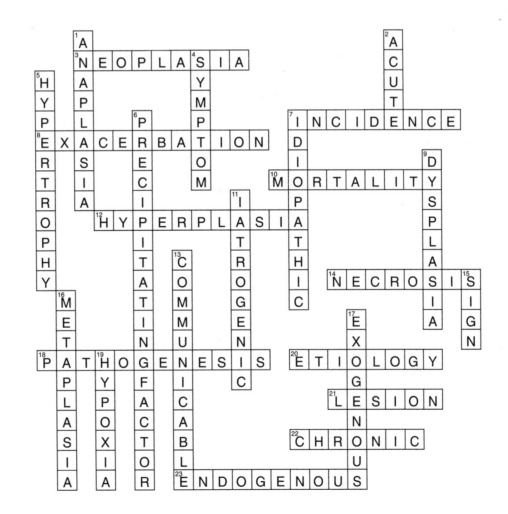

Inflammation and Healing

1. (p. 20) mechanical barrier such as intact skin and mucous membrane
2. (p. 20)
   second: processes of phagocytosis and inflammation
   third: the immune system
3. (p. 20) The immune system is the specific defense mechanism of the body. It provides protection by stimulating a unique response following exposure to foreign substances. (See also review of the immune system in Chapter 3.)
4. (p. 20 and Fig. 2-2, p. 21) Process by which neutrophils and macrophages engulf and destroy bacteria, cellular debris, or foreign material. Neutrophils and monocytes are circulating in the blood and enter the interstitial fluid when inflammation occurs. Macrophages are located (fixed) in tissues such as the alveoli, liver, and spleen.
5. (p. 23) Transient vasoconstriction is followed by vasodilation, hyperemia, and increased capillary permeability in response to chemical mediator (e.g., histamine, serotonin, etc.) released at the site of injury. This allows for the accumulation in the area of fluid (to dilute any toxic substances) and specific plasma proteins such as globulins or antibodies (to react with specific antigens) and fibrinogen (to form a fibrin mesh to localize the problem).
6. (p. 24)
   • redness due to vasodilation in the injured area

• warmth due to hyperemia or increased blood flow to the area
• swelling or edema due to the shift of protein and fluid into the interstitial space
• pain resulting from increased fluid pressure on nerve endings and the irritation caused by chemical mediators
• loss of function if cells lack nutrients or if swelling interferes with joint movement

7. (p. 23)
   Events of the cellular response
   • chemotaxis
   • margination
   • emigration (diapedesis)
   • phagocytosis and subsequent release of lysosomal enzymes
8. (Table 2-2, p. 24)
   a. vii
   b. iii
   c. ii
   d. i
   e. vii and viii
   f. vi
   g. vi
   h. i, iv, vi
9. (pp. 24-25) Fever due to the release of pyrogens by leukocytes and macrophages; malaise, fatigue, headache, and anorexia.
10. (pp. 22-25 and Fig. 2-5, p. 27)

Characteristic	Acute Inflammation	Chronic Inflammation
Causative agents	Direct damage (trauma) Chemicals Ischemia Cell necrosis or infarction Allergic reactions Physical agents (burns) Foreign bodies (splinters or dirt) Infection	When the cause persists and is not removed or eradicated
Onset of symptoms	Immediate Delayed (e.g., sunburn)	Delayed
Intensity of symptoms	Severity varies with the situation or cause	Varies depending on the cause and pathophysiology and duration
Duration	Usually of short duration but may be prolonged	Prolonged
Cells involved	Neutrophils and macrophages; lymphocytes if an immune response involved.	Lymphocytes, macrophages, and fibroblasts
Outcome	Healing unless it becomes chronic due to persistence of causative agent; regeneration; or resolution	Scarring and/or granuloma

11. (p. 30)

R = Rest allows time for healing, minimizing further pain and irritation to the injured area

I = Early application of cold causes vasoconstriction, decreasing pain and edema

C = Compression to facilitate blood clotting, prevent or minimize excess fluid accumulation

E = Elevation improves fluid flow away from the damaged area

12. (p. 30) heat, physiotherapy, adequate nutrition and hydration, mild to moderate exercise, elastic stockings to reduce fluid accumulation

13. (Table 2-4, p. 29) NSAIDs are analgesic and antipyretic. They may cause allergic reactions, slow blood clotting, and cause nausea and/or stomach ulceration. Steroids decrease immune responses and increase the risk of infection, blood pressure, and edema. They may also cause osteoporosis and skeletal muscle wasting.

14. (Table 2-4, p. 29-30) NSAIDs are anti-inflammatory. They may cause allergic reactions and slow blood clotting. Acetaminophen has no anti-inflammatory action. High doses may cause kidney and liver damage.

15. (p. 31) Resolution occurs when there is minimal tissue damage, the damage is repaired, and cells recover and resume normal function in a short time. Regeneration is the healing process that occurs in tissues whose cells are capable of mitosis (e.g., epithelial cells of the skin, gastrointestinal tract). The damaged cells are replaced by the proliferation of nearby undamaged cells.

16. (p. 33)

i. Inoperable bullet wound to the brain may be inaccessible without further tissue damage and loss of function.

ii. Malnutrition, especially deficiencies in vitamins such as C, E, and K, would impair the blood-clotting capability of the individual, impairing wound closure and repair of damaged tissues.

iii. Large, deep cuts, for example, especially if untreated, or presenting difficult suture closure would facilitate extensive scar formation; e.g., cuts due to broken glass or power tools.

iv. Anticlotting medications would limit or impair clotting and hence wound closure; e.g., aspirin and other blood-thinning drugs prior to surgery.

v. Nutritional status is often inadequate in the elderly, and the aging process itself slows down normal healing responses at many levels.

vi. Foreign bodies, if not removed, impair wound closure and promote scarring as well as predispose to infection; e.g., a large splinter.

vii. If the blood supply is limited or cut off from the damaged tissue, then most of the cellular and blood factors necessary for healing would not reach the affected area; e.g., a thrombus or an embolus.

viii. Infection requires its own cure, before healing can occur; removal of the infectious agent, if impaired or delayed, would prolong the healing process, leading to more extensive scarring and, if untreated, perhaps systemic infection. A puncture wound, like a rusty nail, could bring infection to the damaged tissue. Another example is a bite from a rabid animal.

ix. Broken bones, if not immobilized, do not heal properly.

x. Disease, if chronic and with systemic effects, could impair immune and other normal healing tissue responses. Diabetes, for example, may result in impaired circulation to the damaged area.

17. (pp. 30-31) loss of function; contractures and obstructions; adhesions; hypertrophic scar tissue; ulceration

18. (pp. 35-36; Fig. 2-10, p. 36; Fig. 2-11, p. 37)

i. The percentage of body surface area (BSA) burned, using the "rule of nines" for calculation to determine extent of injury and fluid replacement needs (Fig. 2-12, p. 38)

ii. Partial-thickness burns involve the epidermis and part of the dermis; deep partial-thickness burns involve destruction of the epidermis and part of the dermis; full-thickness burns result in destruction of all skin layers and often underlying subcutaneous tissues as well.

19. (p. 35) Nerves in the burned area have been destroyed.

20. (p. 33; see Fig. 2-9, p. 35):

i. hypertrophic scar formation due to excess collagen deposits leading to hard, often elevated, ridges of scar tissue

ii. a thick coagulated crust that develops following a full-thickness burn (p. 35)

iii. narrowing of structures (p. 33)

iv. bands of scar tissue joining two surfaces that are normally separate (p. 33)

v. a surface lesion due to breakdown of surface tissue

vi. interstitial fluid accumulation in an area of inflammation (p. 24)

vii. contracture: fixation and deformity of a joint as a result of scar formation and shrinkage (p. 33)

CHAPTER 3

Immunity and Abnormal Responses

1. (p. 46 and Chapters 1 and 2)

Inflammation is a nonspecific body defense response to any tissue injury, which may be caused by chemical, physical agents, trauma, etc.; it involves neutrophils and macrophages as part of the cellular response and chemical mediators like histamine and prostaglandins with various biologic effects.

Immunity is a specific host defense response to "foreign" (nonself) antigens; it involves specific cellular (T and B lymphocytes) and humoral (antibodies) components and mediators (e.g., comple-

155

ment); and it varies depending on the nature of the antigenic stimulus (immediate and delayed hypersensitivities).

2. (pp. 46-47) A cell surface antigen is a unique protein or glycoprotein configuration that is a distinctive marker for the recognition of a cell by the immune system. They provide the means by which the immune system distinguishes self from nonself. It is important because it provides for the detection and identification of "nonself" by the immune system. This differentiation underlies the host defense against infection and other foreign antigens, and it forms the basis for selection of compatible organs and tissues for transplantation.

3. (pp. 46-47) HLAs are the major histocompatibility complex (MHC) cell membrane antigens on human leukocytes that determine "self" and serve as the basis for identifying histocompatible cells and tissues for transplantation, including blood transfusion. These antigens representing "self" are present on an individual's cell membranes.

4. (Table 3-1, p. 48, and Chapter 2, Table 2-1, p. 23)

Chemical Mediator	Source	Effects
Histamine	Mast cells and basophils	Vasodilation and increased vascular permeability, contraction of bronchiolar smooth muscle; pruritis
Prostaglandins	Group of lipids synthesized in mast cells	Various effects from causing inflammation, vasodilation, increased capillary permeability, and pain
Cytokines (lymphokines, monokines, interleukins, interferon)	T-lymphocytes and macrophages	Increase in plasma proteins, ESR; Stimulate activation and proliferation of B and T cells and communication between cells (messengers); induce fever, leukocytosis, and chemotaxis
Leukotrienes	Group of lipids derived from mast cells and basophils	Contraction of bronchiolar smooth muscle; vasodilation and increased capillary permeability; chemotaxis
Kinins (bradykinin)	Activation of plasma protein (kinogen; e.g., bradykinin)	Vasodilation, edema, and pain
Complement	Group of proteins circulating in the bloodstream; activated by antigen-antibody reactions on cell surface	Release of chemical mediators, promoting inflammation, chemotaxis, phagocytosis, cell membrane damage (e.g., hemolysis)

5. (Table 3-1, p. 48, and see also Table 2-1, p. 23)
   i. histamine, prostaglandins, kinins, leukotrienes
   ii. histamine, prostaglandins, leukotrienes
   iii. cytokines, leukotrienes, complement
   iv. prostaglandins, kinins
   v. histamine, leukotrienes
   vi. cytokines
   vii. histamine
   viii. TNF, cytokines

6. (Table 3-1, p. 48)
   macrophages: phagocytosis; foreign antigen recognition
   natural killer (NK) cells: destroy foreign cells, virus-infected cells, and cancer cells
   T-lymphocytes
      cytotoxic or killer T cells: destroy antigens and cancer and virus-infected cells
      helper T cells (T4 or CD4): activate B and T cells; limit immune response

   memory T cells: remember antigen and stimulate immune response upon subsequent exposure (secondary response)
   suppressor T cells (T8): limit immune response
   B-lymphocytes
      plasma cells: produce specific antibody
      B memory cells: secondary antibody response

7. (Table 3-1, p. 48) monocytes, macrophages, basophils

8. (Table 3-1, p. 48) helper T cells

9. (Table 3-2, p. 50)
   IgG: primary and secondary antibody responses; activates complement; includes antibacterial, antivirals, and antitoxins; crosses placenta, creates passive immunity in newborns
   IgM: primary antibody responses; activates complement; forms natural antibodies; involved in blood ABO incompatibility reactions

IgA: found in secretions such as tears and saliva, in mucous membranes, and in colostrum to provide protection for newborns

IgE: binds to mast cells in skin and mucous membranes; when linked to allergen, causes release of histamine and other chemicals, resulting in inflammation

IgD: attached to B cells; activates B cells

10. (p. 50) Antibodies exert their effect by binding to the specific antigen that elicited their production, usually on a cell or bacterial surface, resulting in antigen destruction, cell membrane damage (especially in the presence of complement), and, in the case of red blood cells, cell lysis. Some antigen-antibody-complement complexes are also chemotactic, attracting phagocytes and other cells to the site.

11. (p. 51) Primary response on initial antigen exposure may range from days to weeks. Secondary response is almost immediate.

12. (Fig. 3-3, p. 52) Primary response is approximately 3 to 4 weeks. Secondary response is quicker with much higher titer within a week or two.

13. (p. 53) to promote a stronger, faster secondary immune response

14. (p. 51) There are many strains of a virus or bacteria that cause a disease, and they may mutate readily, causing new strains, then, because the immune response is specific, infection with one strain does not create immunity to subsequent exposures to new, different strains.

15. (pp. 51-52; Table 3-3)

Characteristic	Active Immunity	Passive Immunity
Method of acquiring	Exposure to an antigen and production of specific antibodies	Receiving specific antibody passively (i.e., produced by others who have been exposed to the antigens) via either milk (newborn infants) or injection of pooled IgG fractions
Onset of immunity	Several weeks for a primary response	Immediate upon receipt of the antibodies
Duration of effectiveness	Depending on the nature of the antigen, usually lasts for years (memory T cells)	Months
Examples	Polio, measles, diphtheria, vaccines, chickenpox	Breast milk, rabies immune globulin and snake antivenom serum

16. (p. 55) A close match of HLAs between donor and host tissues reduces risk of rejection. The common treatment involves immunosuppressive drugs such as cyclosporine, azathioprine (Imuran), and prednisone.

17. (p. 55) The term *opportunistic* describes micro-organisms that are usually harmless in healthy individuals; however, patients taking immuno-suppressant drugs have limited body defenses.

18. (p. 66) Preventative antibiotics are usually administered because opportunistic infections are common and can be difficult to treat. They are best prevented.

19. (Table 3-5, p. 55)

Type	Mechanism	Effects	Example
I	IgE bound to mast cells; release of histamine and chemical mediators	Immediate inflammation and pruritis	Hay fever; anaphylaxis
II	IgG or IgM reacts with antigen on cell—complement activated	Cell lysis and phagocytosis	ABO blood incompatibility
III	Antigen-antibody complex deposits in tissue—complement activated	Inflammation; vasculitis	Autoimmune disorders: SLE; glomerulonephritis
IV	Antigen binds to T-lymphocyte; sensitizing lymphocytes that releases lymphokines	Delayed inflammation	Contact dermatitis; transplant rejection

20. (pp. 56-58, Fig. 3-6) (see also Chapter 18)

	Hypovolemic Shock (Chapter 18)	**Anaphylactic Shock (pp. 56–58, Fig. 3-6)**
Etiology	Hemorrhage, severe burns, dehydration, peritonitis, pancreatitis	Severe, life-threatening, systemic hypersensitivity (allergic) reaction caused by insect stings, ingestion of nuts or shellfish, penicillin or local anesthetics
Distinguishing features	Anxiety, restlessness, thirst early; tachycardia, cool, pale, moist skin, oliguria, hyperventilation during compensation. Progressive: lethargy, weakness, faintness; metabolic acidosis; CNS depression; organ damage	Very rapid onset of decreased blood pressure, weakness, fainting; itching; airway obstruction, cough, dyspnea; edema around the face, hands and feet; hives, urticaria, fear and panic. If untreated, collapse and loss of consciousness
Specific treatment	Patient put in supine position; cover to keep warm; call for help or transport to hospital. Administer oxygen if available.	Epinephrine injection immediately; oxygen administration; antihistamine injection; treatment for shock; summon help/transport to hospital; CPR, if necessary

21. (p. 59) antihistamine drugs for early signs and symptoms; glucocorticoids for severe or prolonged reactions

22. (pp. 61-62 and Fig. 3-10, p. 63) when individuals develop antibodies to their own cells or cellular material

23. (p. 64) prednisone (glucocorticoid) to reduce the immune response and subsequent inflammation; hydroxychloroquine (antimalarial) may be used to reduce exacerbations

24. (p. 64) SLE is diagnosed by the presence of numerous ANAs, especially anti-DNA, as well as other antibodies. Lupus erythematous (LE) cells are mature neutrophils containing nuclear material, found in the circulating blood and are a positive sign.

25. (Table 3-7, p. 64)
    i. skin: butterfly rash
    ii. joints: polyarthritis
    iii. heart: carditis and pericarditis
    iv. blood vessels: Raynaud's phenomenon
    v. blood: anemia, leukopenia, thrombocytopenia
    vi. kidneys: glomerulonephritis, with marked proteinuria and progressive damage
    vii. lungs: pleurisy
    viii. central nervous system: psychosis, depression, mood changes, seizures

26. (p. 64) usually treated by a rheumatologist with prednisone, nonsteroidal anti-inflammatory drugs, and hydroxychloroquine for exacerbations

27. (p. 65, Table 3-8)
    primary: hypogammaglobulinemia; thymic aplasia, DiGeorge's syndrome, CIDS, inherited deficits in any one or more of the components
    secondary: kidney disease, Hodgkin's disease, AIDS, radiation, immunosuppressive drugs, immunosuppression, malnutrition

28. (p. 66) predisposition to opportunistic infections and an increased risk of cancer

29. (p. 66) prophylactic antimicrobials to reduce incidence of opportunistic infections; gamma globulin replacement therapy

30. (pp. 66-67) Human immunodeficiency virus (HIV) is the causative agent for AIDS. It is a "slow-acting" retrovirus containing two strands of RNA and the enzyme reverse transcriptase. Its envelope is characterized by spikes of glycoprotein. The virus is inactivated by many disinfectants and high temperatures.

31. (pp. 68-69) HIV must enter the bloodstream of the recipient through transmission of body fluids such as blood, semen, and vaginal secretions. Transmission most often occurs through unprotected sexual intercourse with an HIV-positive partner, intravenous injection with contaminated needles, maternal-fetal transmission, and blood transfusion

32. (p. 69) At the highest risk are intravenous drug users, people with multiple sexual partners, and the unborn fetuses of HIV-positive mothers.

33. (pp. 67-68, see also Figures 3-13 and 3-14) Infected individuals usually become HIV positive within 2 to 10 weeks, but the "window" may be as long as 6 months. Full-blown AIDS may not occur for many years. After an initial infection, mild "flu-like" symptoms appear in 3 to 6 weeks, followed by an asymptomatic latent period that may last for years before phase 3, acute onset of signs and symptoms, including multiple severe opportunistic infections and rare cancers such as Kaposi's sarcoma.

34. (p. 68) A blood test is performed for HIV antibodies. A positive test is followed by the Western blot test. The "window period" refers to the time from infection to the presence of HIV antibodies. This may be anywhere from 2 weeks to 6 months depending on the mode of transmission.

35. (Fig. 3-13, p. 67) Full-blown AIDS may not occur for 6 to 7 years on average.

36. (p. 69, Fig. 3-14, p. 68) AIDS is diagnosed by a major decrease in the CD4 T-helper lymphocyte count and a change in the CD4⁺-to-CD8⁺ ratio in the presence of opportunistic infection or certain cancers.

37. (p. 67) Helper T4 lymphocytes are the major target and, when destroyed, eliminate the immune surveillance and detection function of these cells, thereby interfering with their critical function in the initiation of both humoral and cellular immunity.

38. (Fig. 3-14, p. 68; pp. 69-70) mild, self-limited nonspecific "flu-like" symptoms: low fever, fatigue, joint pain, and sore throat

39. (pp. 69-71)
   i. generalized effects: lymphadenopathy, fatigue and weakness, headache, and arthralgia
   ii. opportunistic infections (see also gastrointestinal manifestations): *Pneumocystis carinii* in the lungs, causing severe pneumonia; herpes simplex, causing cold sores; and *Candida,* a fungus infection of the mouth and esophagus
   iii. gastrointestinal manifestations, including parasitic infections: chronic severe diarrhea, vomiting, and ulcers; necrotizing periodontal disease; severe weight loss, malnutrition and wasting
   iv. oral manifestations: cold sores (herpes simplex) and *Candida*
   v. respiratory manifestations: *Pneumocystis carinii* causing pneumonia
   vi. nervous system manifestations: HIV encephalopathy (AIDS dementia), aggravated by lymphomas, causing confusion, progressive cognitive impairment, memory loss, loss of coordination and balance, and depression; seizures
   vii. malignancies: Kaposi's sarcoma and non-Hodgkin's lymphomas

40. (p. 72) antiviral drugs such as AZT; protease inhibitors; viral integrase inhibitors such as saquinavir and ritonavir; reverse transcriptase inhibitors such as zidovudine and lamivudine; various drug combinations known as "cocktails"; prophylactic medications include antibacterial, antifungal, and antituberculosis drugs; other drugs such as antidiarrheals (e.g., Imodium) and vitamin and mineral supplements may be required

41. (p. 72) Prognosis is much improved due to earlier detection and newer drug and nutritional therapies. Without treatment, death occurs within several years of diagnosis.

CHAPTER 4

Infection

1. (Chapter 2, p. 20; Chapter 4, p. 78) Inflammation is a normal body response. It is the second line of defense caused by anything that results in tissue damage. Infection is caused by pathogenic microorganisms.

2. (pp. 78-79, Fig. 4-1)
   bacilli: *Clostridium tetani*
   cocci: *Staphylococcus aureus*
   spirals: *Treponema pallidum*

3. (Fig. 4-3, pp. 79-80) The basic structure of a bacterium consists of an outer rigid cell wall, a cell membrane, a DNA strand, and cytoplasm. In addition, some species contain an external capsule or slime layer, specialized structures such as flagellae, and pili or fimbriae.

4. (p. 81) Exotoxins are produced/secreted by gram-positive bacteria. Endotoxins are components of the cell wall of gram-negative organisms.

5. (p. 81, Fig. 4-1, p. 82) Endospores are latent forms of some bacterial species with an outer coat that is resistant to heat and other environmental conditions. The process of spore formation is illustrated in Figure 4-4, p. 82. Examples of spore-producing bacteria include tetanus *(C. tetani)* and botulism *(C. botulinum).*

6. (p. 81, Fig. 4-1, p. 82) Binary fission is simply dividing in half, forming two daughter cells identical to the parent bacterium.

7. (Table 4-2, p. 84)

	Bacterial Cells	**Human Cells**
Cell wall	Present	Not present
Cell membrane	Present—selectively permeable; site of metabolic processes	Present—selectively permeable
Capsule or slime coat	Present in some	Not present
Flagella	Present	Sperm only
Pili or fimbriae	Present in some	Not present
Cilia	Not present	Present in some
Membrane-bound organelles (mitochondria, Golgi complex lysosomes, endoplasmic reticulum)	Not present	Present
Ribosomes	Present	Present—larger
Nucleus	Not present	Present
Number of chromosomes	Single; circular	46; paired (except sex cells)
Method of reproduction	Binary fission	Mitosis

8. (p. 81) They require a living host cell for replication.
9. (p. 81) The virion consists of a protein coat or capsid and a DNA or RNA nucleic acid core.
10. (Fig. 4-5, p. 83) Virus attaches to the host cell and penetrates. It uncoats and takes over the host cell DNA. The host cell synthesizes viral components. The components assemble and are released by host cell lysis.
11. (p. 85, see also Fig. 4-1, p. 78) Fungi are classified as eukaryotic. They consist of cells or chains of cells and may have long filaments called hyphae that intertwine to form a mass called the mycelium, which is large enough to be visible.
12. (Table 4-2, p. 84)

	Bacteria	**Fungus**	**Virus**
Structure	Cell wall, cell membrane, cytoplasm, DNA	Cell wall, hyphae Eukaryotic	Capsid, nucleic acid core of either RNA or DNA
Method of reproduction	Binary fission	Budding, spores, extending hyphae	Use host cell to replicate and assemble components
Method of culturing	Various culture media	Culture media (simple glucose/agar)	Living host cells
Drugs used to treat	Antimicrobials	Antifungal agents	Antiviral drugs

13. (pp. 84-85)
    i. chlamydiae: pelvic inflammatory disease; eye infections in newborn of infected mothers
    ii. rickettsiae: typhus; Rocky Mountain spotted fever
    iii. mycoplasmas: pneumonia
    iv. protozoa: *Trichomonas vaginalis;* malaria; amebic dysentery
14. (p. 87) a worm
15. (p. 88) microorganisms that normally inhabit various areas of the body such as the skin and gastrointestinal tract
16. (p. 89) lungs, bladder, and stomach

17. (p. 91)
Virulence is the degree of pathogenicity of a microbe or pathogen. It can be enhanced by production of exotoxins or endotoxins, destructive enzymes, spore formation, and presence of bacterial capsule.
Pathogenicity is the capacity of a microbe to cause disease. Immunodeficiency or immunodepression can result in opportunistic infections; relocation of normal flora to another body site can also result in their production of disease.
18. (pp. 79-88)
    i. *Pneumocystis carinii* pneumonia: fungus
    ii. candidiasis: fungus

iii. syphilis: bacteria
   iv. trichomoniasis: protozoa
    v. tuberculosis: bacteria
   vi. pneumonia: bacteria; viruses; fungi, myco-plasma
  vii. tetanus: bacteria
 viii. Rocky Mountain spotted fever: rickettsia
   ix. tinea pedis: fungus
    x. herpes simplex: virus
   xi. influenza: virus
  xii. botulism: bacteria
19. (pp. 92-95, Fig. 4-10, p. 93) The infectious cycle is the sequence or chain of events that lead to infection and disease by a pathogen. The components and means to break the cycle include:
   locating and removing the reservoir or sources of infection
   blocking the exit from the source; providing or cleaning/sterilizing barriers
   maintaining immunizations
   treating or quarantining infection or carrier
20. (p. 97) to take a tissue culture of a specimen that is placed in a medium containing various antimicrobials to determine the nature and drug sensitivity of the microbe
21. (pp. 96-97, Table 4-5, p. 96) Microbes are present at the source of infection. With infection due to bacteria, purulent exudate (pus) and tissue necrosis usually develop at the site. Lymphadenopathy, high temperature, and leukocytosis are often present. Inflammation results in a serous exudate and milder systemic effects.
22.   i. antibacterial spectrum (p. 98): The range of bacteria for which the drug is effective: narrow, either gram positive or negative; broad, both gram-positive and -negative bacteria
     ii. bacterial resistance (pp. 97-98): bacteria that develop or adapt in order to lose their sensitivity to a drug such as altering their metabolism to block the drug's effects, producing enzymes that inactivate the drug, altering their cell membranes
    iii. bactericidal (p. 98): drugs that destroy microorganisms
     iv. bacteriostatic (p. 98): drugs that reduce the rate of bacterial reproduction
23. (p. 99) Because viruses are obligate intracellular parasites, a drug that destroys viruses would also destroy the host cell.

24. (p. 99) allergic reaction—anaphylaxis
25. (p. 98) a secondary infection by pathogens that results from disruption or reduction of the normal resident flora by antimicrobial drugs
26. (p. 98) A superinfection occurs only during treatment with antimicrobial agents. An opportunistic infection occurs in an individual with decreased immunity. Both are usually caused by fungi that are part of the normal resident flora.
27. (pp. 97-98) when the identity of the bacterium is known; after culture and sensitivity have been completed
28. (p. 98) The drug prevents replication of the bacteria, thereby keeping the number of bacteria constant—the body's own defensive cells will destroy the organism.
29. (p. 98) if the individual was immunosuppressed (e.g., organ transplant recipient) or immunodeficient (e.g., someone with AIDS)
30. (pp. 97-98) Bacteria adapt and/or mutate to develop various means of losing drug sensitivity; excessive or unnecessary use of drugs provides a stimulus for such adaptation.
31. (p. 98) because they may reduce the risk of secondary bacterial infection
32. (p. 98) Drug should be taken regularly according to the prescription. Drug should be taken until the prescription is completely used. Follow instructions regarding food or fluid intake. Provide a good medical history including known drug allergies.

CHAPTER 5

Neoplasms

 1. (p. 107)
     i. neoplasm: a tumor, a cellular growth that is no longer responding to normal body controls
    ii. benign: tumor of differentiated cells that reproduce at higher than normal rate but do not spread
   iii. malignant: tumor of undifferentiated, nonfunctional cells that reproduce rapidly, infiltrate surrounding areas, and may spread away as metastases to other organs and tissues
    iv. carcinoma: malignant tumors of epithelial tissue
     v. sarcoma: malignant tumors of connective tissue
    vi. anaplasia: growth of undifferentiated cells of varying size and shape (p. 109)

2. (p. 107, Table 5-1)

	Benign Tumor	**Malignant Tumor**
Pancreas	Adenoma	Adenocarcinoma
Fat	Lipoma	Liposarcoma
Bone	Osteoma	Osteosarcoma
Liver	Hepatoma	Hepatocarcinoma
Cartilage	Chondroma	Chondrosarcoma
Skin	Epithelioma	Carcinoma; melanoma

3. (pp. 107-108, Table 5-2 [modified], p. 108)

	Benign Tumors	**Malignant Tumors**
CELL GROWTH Shape Size Nucleus Differentiation Mitosis Antigenic properties Cohesiveness	Similar to normal cells Similar to normal cells Similar to normal cells Differentiated Fairly normal Unaltered Remain localized	Varied Varied Large Undifferentiated Atypical and increased Altered surface antigens Cells not adhesive, can infiltrate tissue
GROWTH RATE	Relatively slow	Rapid
PRESENCE OF CAPSULE	Frequently encapsulated	No capsule
SPREAD	Locally	Locally invasive and spreads to other sites by bloodstream or lymphatics
SYSTEMIC EFFECTS	Rare	Common, widespread
LIFE THREATENING	Seldom unless in vital areas such as the brain	Life threatening

4. (p. 109)
   i. compression of blood vessels: ischemia, necrosis, and areas of inflammation around the tumor; potential for infection
   ii. compression or obstruction of a tube or duct: blockage of secretion or normal flow of air (bronchi), food (GI tract), blood, or lymph depending on location
   iii. compression of nerves: pain and loss of function
   iv. erosion of blood vessels and other structures: hemorrhage, inflammation, necrosis
   v. invasion and replacement of normal tissue: loss of normal tissue function

5. (p. 110)
   i. weight loss and cachexia: anorexia, fatigue, pain, stress, nutrient trapping, altered metabolism, and cachectic factors produced by macrophages
   ii. anemia: anorexia, decreased appetite and food intake, chronic bleeding, and bone marrow depression

   iii. systemic infections: host resistance decline; tissue breakdown and diminished immune system function; immobility
   iv. bleeding: local invasion/erosion of blood vessels by tumor; bone marrow depression, and hypoproteinemia

6. (p. 110) additional problems associated with certain tumors: e.g., bronchogenic carcinoma cells producing ACTH, causing manifestations of Cushing's syndrome

7. (p. 109) Unusual bleeding or discharge anywhere in the body; change in bowel or bladder habits (e.g., prolonged diarrhea or discomfort); a change in a wart or mole (i.e., color, size, or shape); a sore that does not heal (on the skin or in the mouth, anywhere); unexplained weight loss; anemia or low hemoglobin, and persistent fatigue; persistent cough or hoarseness without reason; a solid lump, often painless, in the breast or testes or anywhere on the body

8. (p. 111)
    i. medical history: reveal family history and evidence of the warning signs of cancer
    ii. physical examination: identification of painful areas, palpable lumps and masses
    iii. x-ray, ultrasound, magnetic resonance imaging (MRI), and computed tomography (CT or CAT scan): signs of abnormal growth or changes in organs and tissues
    iv. tumor markers: tumor-specific enzymes, antigens, or hormones that can be detected by tests of blood and bodily fluids, e.g., CEA, hCG, PSA
    v. biopsy and histological and cytological examinations: histopathological confirmation of diagnosis of malignancy
9. (p. 111) Malignant tumor cells lack cohesiveness and easily separate from the growing tumor mass; if invasive and eroding blood or lymphatic vessels, tumor cells can enter the circulation and reach distant sites. This is called metastasis.
10. (pp. 112-113)
    Grading is a reflection of the degree of differentiation or undifferentiation (degree of malignancy) of the tumor cells. Staging is the classification of tumors that reflects the extent of disease, i.e., size of primary tumor, extent of lymph node spread, and metastasis (as in breast cancer).
11. (p. 115; see also Fig. 5-8, p. 116) Initiating factors cause the first irreversible cellular changes in the process of carcinogenesis. Promoters cause additional changes in DNA, resulting in less differentiation and greater rate of mitosis.
12. (Table 5-4, p. 117)
    genetic factors: high family incidence of breast cancers
    viruses: hepatitis virus; hepatic cancer
    radiation: skin cancer
    chemical exposure: lung cancer
    chronic irritation or inflammation: ulcerative colitis—colon cancer
    increasing age: many cancers are more common
    diet: high-fat diet—colon cancer
    hormones: estrogen—endometrial cancer
13. (pp. 117-122) Radiation, surgery, and chemotherapy are often used in combination to completely eradicate local tumor and treat and/or prevent metastases.
14. (p. 117)
    curative: complete eradication of tumor, usually localized and small at time of diagnosis; e.g., surgery (including laser) for skin cancer

palliative: in advanced cancer, intended to reduce the manifestations and complications and provide some quality of life for terminal patients; e.g., surgery to remove a tumor to relieve pain and pressure on surrounding tissues
prophylactic: prevention of metastasis; e.g., chemotherapy and radiation after surgery for breast cancer
15. (p. 119) Radiation causes mutations in the tumor cell DNA, preventing mitosis and tumor growth and causing immediate cell death; it also damages blood vessels, cutting off tumor blood supply.
16. (p. 120, Fig. 5-10, p. 121) antimitotics, antimetabolites, alkylating agents, and some antibiotics that interfere with protein synthesis and DNA replication at different stages of the cell cycle
17. (p. 120) Radiation and chemotherapy are most effective against reproducing cells, both normal and malignant because of their affects on DNA replication. Therefore, normal cells that are dividing regularly are at the greatest risk: e.g., skin, GI tract mucosa, bone marrow, and gonads. Adverse effects include bone marrow depression (resulting in anemia, infections, bleeding, etc.), nausea and vomiting, and hair loss.
18. (p. 122) Biologic response modifiers are agents that augment the natural immune response to improve immune surveillance and destruction of "foreign" tumor cells.
19. (p. 122) Glucocorticoids may be prescribed to decrease mitosis and increase erythrocyte count; improve appetite and sense of well-being, and also decrease inflammation and swelling around the tumor.
20. (p. 122) sex hormones when the tumor cells are hormone responsive; hormone blocking agents for tumors that depend on hormones for growth; angiogenesis inhibitor to prevent enhanced blood supply to tumors; analgesics for pain management
21. (p. 123) basal cell carcinoma
22. (p. 66) Malignant tumors often have altered, "nonself" antigens on their surface, which, if detected early, may invoke an immune response that prevents the growth and spread of the tumor. If the immune system is compromised or deficient (e.g., AIDS), then transformed cells go undetected until sufficient growth has occurred to establish the tumor.

23. answer to crossword puzzle

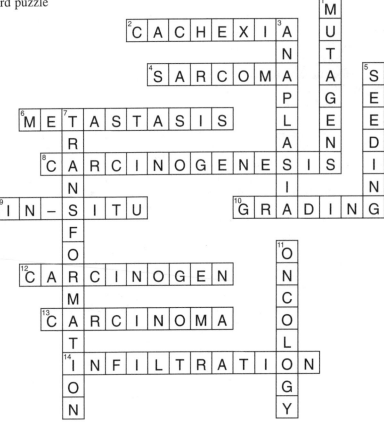

CHAPTER 6

Fluid, Electrolyte, and Acid-Base Imbalances

1. (p. 133) excess fluid in the interstitial compartment
2. (pp. 133-135, Fig. 6-2)
   1. increased capillary hydrostatic pressure, forcing excessive amounts of fluid out and prevents return of fluid from the interstitial compartment
   2. loss of plasma proteins, reducing plasma osmotic pressure
   3. obstruction of lymphatic circulation, restricting the return of excess fluid and protein to the general circulation
   4. increased capillary permeability—as in inflammation, resulting in fluid and protein movement into the interstitial compartment
3. (pp. 133-135)
   i. obstruction of lymphatic circulation due to removal of lymphatic vessels; increased capillary permeability and increased capillary hydrostatic pressure immediately following surgery
   ii. loss of plasma proteins due to decreased production of plasma proteins
   iii. increased capillary hydrostatic pressure and increased capillary permeability
   iv. increased capillary hydrostatic pressure due to increased blood volume; possibly due to decreased capillary osmotic pressure due to protein-wasting kidney disease
   v. increased capillary hydrostatic pressure due to effects of gravity
   vi. increased capillary hydrostatic pressure and increased capillary permeability due to inflammation
   vii. obstruction of lymphatic circulation or increased capillary hydrostatic pressure if blood vessels are compressed
   viii. increased capillary permeability and loss of plasma proteins
   ix. increased capillary hydrostatic pressure due to increased water retention
   x. loss of plasma proteins due to decreased synthesis of plasma proteins
   xi. increased capillary hydrostatic pressure
   xii. increased capillary hydrostatic pressure and increased capillary permeability due to inflammation
4. (p. 154, Think About)
   i. diuretic
   ii. glucocorticoid
   iii. nonsteroidal anti-inflammatory
   iv. antihistamine
   v. adrenergic agonist or sympathomimetic—epinephrine
   vi. antibiotic
5. (pp. 135-136, Table 6-3)
   local swelling
   pale, gray or red skin color

weight gain with pitting edema

functional impairment of joints or movement of organs such as the heart and lungs

slow, bounding pulse and high blood pressure

pulmonary congestion, cough, rales

lethargy, possible seizures

pain

impairment of arterial circulation

6. (p. 136)

vomiting

diarrhea

excessive sweating

diabetic ketoacidosis

insufficient water intake

fever

drainage or suction

severe burns

decreased aldosterone or ADH secretion

prolonged hyperventilation

7. (Table 6-3, pp. 135-137) Manifestations include sunken, soft eyes; decreased skin turgor; thirst, weight loss; rapid, weak pulse and low blood pressure; fatigue, weakness, dizziness, and possible stupor; increased body temperature. The most serious complication of dehydration is hypovolemic shock.

8. (p. 137) Compensatory mechanisms include increasing thirst, increasing heart rate, constricting cutaneous blood vessels, and decreasing urinary output.

9. (pp. 137-146)

i. hyponatremia, hyperkalemia, hypocalcemia, hypermagnesemia, hyperphosphatemia

ii. hyponatremia, hypochloremia

iii. hypernatremia, hyperchloremia

iv. hypernatremia, hypokalemia, hyperchloremia

v. hypercalcemia, hypophosphatemia, hypomagnesemia

vi. hyponatremia, hypochloremia

vii. hypercalcemia

viii. hyponatremia, hypokalemia, hypomagnesemia (with potassium-sparing diuretics: hyperkalemia)

ix. hyponatremia, hyperkalemia, hypochloremia

x. hypocalcemia

xi. hypercalcemia

xii. hyponatremia, hypokalemia, hypophosphatemia

10. (p. 144) skeletal muscle spasm due to hypocalcemia

11. (Table 6-6, p. 143) hypokalemia and hyperkalemia; (Table 6-8, p. 144) hypocalcemia and hypercalcemia

12. (Table 6-8, p. 144) hypercalcemia

13. (pp. 147-148) Volatile acids can change between liquid and gaseous states. Nonvolatile acids cannot be converted to a gaseous form.

14. (p. 149) 20:1

15. (p. 149) Sodium bicarbonate–carbonic acid system; phosphate system; hemoglobin system; protein system

16. (p. 151, Table 6-9, p. 150) The imbalance is metabolic acidosis. The individual would experience the following manifestations: rapid, deep respirations; lethargy, weakness, confusion; coma; and decreased pH of urine.

17. (Table 6-9, p. 150, and Fig. 6-10, p. 152)

i. metabolic alkalosis—slow, shallow breathing

ii. respiratory acidosis—more acidic urine

iii. metabolic alkalosis—slow, shallow respirations and increased pH of urine

iv. respiratory acidosis—more acidic urine

v. metabolic acidosis—increased rate and depth of respirations and more acidic urine

vi. respiratory alkalosis—period of apnea and increased urine pH

vii. respiratory acidosis—more acidic urine and increased rate and depth of respiration (if possible)

viii. metabolic alkalosis—slow, shallow respirations

ix. metabolic acidosis—increased rate and depth of respirations, more acidic urine

x. metabolic acidosis—increased rate and depth of respiration, more acidic urine

xi. metabolic acidosis—increased rate and depth of respiration

CHAPTER 7

Congenital and Genetic Disorders

1. (pp. 165-166) Inherited disorders are genetic in origin, whereas developmental disorders result from harmful influences occurring during embryonic or fetal development, and may also include premature birth, difficult labor and delivery, and exposure to toxic agents during gestation

2. (pp. 166 and 169) damage to the embryo or fetus by noxious agents such as alcohol, smoke, radiation, narcotics, mercury, some OTC and prescription drugs, and various pathogens such as toxoplasmosis, hepatitis B, mumps, rubeola, varicella, gonorrhea, syphilis, cytomegalovirus, and herpes)

3. (p. 169) The most critical time for development is the first 2 months of gestation, when most of the organogenesis occurs. Poor maternal nutrition means insufficient nutrients for the developing embryo and fetus. Examples of developmental defects resulting from poor nutrition are folic acid deficiency (spina bifida), low iron (anemia), and poor nutrition in general (low birth weight).

4. (p. 170) Difficulties encountered during or after birth that may temporarily deprive the newborn of oxygen can cause brain damage; e.g., cerebral palsy.

5. (pp. 165-166) Inherited disorders are any disorders resulting from abnormalities or damage to the genetic makeup, whereas chromosomal defects usually result from errors during meiosis when the chromosomes are segregating, when the DNA fragments are displaced or lost and therefore could involve many genes.

6. (p. 168) errors in chromosomal duplication or reassembly during meiosis, resulting in abnormal

165

placement of part of a chromosome (translocation), altered structure (deletion), or abnormal number of chromosomes

7. (p. 168, Fig. 7-1, p. 162)
   i. monosomy: when one member of a chromosome pair is lost during meiosis
   ii. trisomy: when there is extra duplication of one member of a chromosome pair, yielding three chromosomes instead of two

8. (p. 168) maternal age over 35

9. (p. 168, Box 7-1, p. 166) Multifactorial disorders occur when a combination of factors is responsible for the congenital disorder; i.e., polygenic, caused by multiple genes or inherited tendency that is expressed following exposure to environmental factors. Examples include anencephaly, cleft lip and palate, clubfoot, etc.

10. (pp. 93, 167) A carrier of an infectious disease is contagious and can pass the infection to others. A carrier of a genetic disorder is heterozygous for that particular disorder and usually does not have any manifestations of the disorder; he may pass the faulty gene on to his children.

11. (pp. 167-168) autosomal recessive and sex-linked recessive disorders

12. (p. 167) heterozygous; does not usually become symptomatic

13. (Fig. 7-4, p. 165)

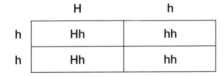

Father

	H	h
h	Hh	hh
h	Hh	hh

   i. father
   ii. 50%
   iii. 0%—there is no carrier state in autosomal dominant disorders; an individual with the faulty gene has the disorder

14. (Fig. 7-4, p. 165)

Father

	H	h
H	HH	Hh
h	Hh	hh

   i. both
   ii. 75%

15. (Fig. 7-4, p. 165)

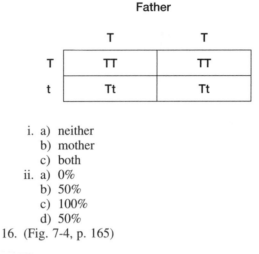

Father

	T	T
T	TT	TT
t	Tt	Tt

   i. a) neither
      b) mother
      c) both
   ii. a) 0%
       b) 50%
       c) 100%
       d) 50%

16. (Fig. 7-4, p. 165)

Father

	T	t
T	TT	Tt
t	Tt	tt

   i. a) neither
      b) both
      c) both
   ii. a) 25%
       b) 50%
       c) 100%
       d) 50%

17. (Fig. 7-4, p. 165)

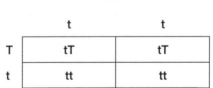

Father

	t	t
T	tT	tT
t	tt	tt

   i. a) father
      b) mother
      c) mother
   ii. a) 50%
       b) 50%
       c) 50%
       d) 50%

18. (p. 167, Fig. 7-4, p. 165)
   i. homozygous
   ii. both
   iii. 25%
   iv. 50%

19. (p. 168, Fig. 7-4, p. 165)

Father

	t	t
t	tt	tt
t	tt	tt

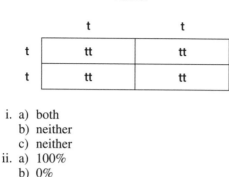

i. a) both
   b) neither
   c) neither
ii. a) 100%
   b) 0%
   c) 0%
   d) 100%

20. (p. 168, Fig.7-4, p. 165)

Square A

	X^H	Y
X^H	$X^H X^H$	$X^H Y$
X^h	$X^h X^H$	$X^h Y$

Square B

	X^h	Y
X^H	$X^H X^h$	$X^H Y$
X^H	$X^H X^h$	$X^H Y$

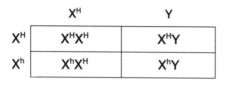

Referring to Square A:
i. a) neither
   b) mother
ii. 25%
iii. male
iv. 25%—female
v. a) 25%
   b) 25%

Referring to Square B:
i. a) father
   b) neither
   c) mother
ii. a) 100%
   b) 0%
   c) 0%
   d) 0%

21. (p. 168, Fig. 7-4, p. 165) There is a 25% chance of a female with the disorder.

	X^h	Y
X^H	$X^H X^h$	$X^H Y$
X^h	$X^h X^h$	$X^h Y$

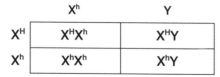

22. (p. 168, Fig. 7-4, p. 165)
   i. $X^d Y$
   ii. mother
   iii. daughter—0%; son—50%
   iv. brother—sex-linked disorder; in order for a female to be affected, father would have the disorder
   v. 50% of sisters will be carriers, 0% of brothers

23. (Box 7-1, p. 166)
   i. multifactorial
   ii. autosomal recessive
   iii. congenital
   iv. autosomal dominant
   v. sex-linked
   vi. autosomal recessive
   vii. X-linked
   viii. chromosomal
   ix. autosomal recessive
   x. autosomal dominant
   xi. autosomal recessive
   xii. multifactorial
   xiii. multifactorial
   xiv. chromosomal

24. (p. 168, Fig. 7-1C, pp. 162, 171) Down syndrome is a chromosomal disorder that is diagnosed prenatally through amniocentesis and karyotyping. The karyotype of an individual with Down syndrome is trisomy 21.

25. (p. 172) Down syndrome is trisomy 21, which results in numerous defects in physical and mental development, including hypotonic muscles, loose joints, cervical instability, delayed developmental states, cognitive impairment, and delayed sexual development. Miscellaneous other conditions may be present, including visual, hearing, and digestive problems; celiac disease, congenital heart disease; decreased resistance to infection; and a high risk of leukemia.

26. (p. 172) Individuals with Down syndrome may have a small head and flat facial profiles, slanted eyes, Brushfield's spots in the irises, mouths that tend to hang open, large protruding tongues and high arched palates, and small hands with single palmar creases.

CHAPTER 8

Adolescence

1. (pp. 179-184)
   a) condition characterized by alternating "binge and purge" behavior; vii. bulimia nervosa
   b) lateral curvature of the spine; iii. scoliosis
   c) extreme weight loss due to self-starvation; vi. anorexia nervosa
   d) exaggerated concave curvature of the lumbar spine; i. lordosis
   e) demineralization of bone; iv. osteoporosis
   f) exaggerated convex curvature of the thoracic spine; ii. kyphosis
   g) bone infection; v. osteomyelitis

2. (p. 150) minor trauma such as a fracture or soft tissue injury; sickle cell anemia
3. (pp. 181-182) The pathophysiology of osteomyelitis includes (1) accumulation of local purulent exudate, which destroys the bone in the damaged area, causing severe pain due to pressure on the nerves; if the fluid pressure is severe, may cause separation of the periosteum; (2) stimulation of surrounding bone development walls off the area; (3) if the periosteum separates due to excess pressure, a sinus may develop, spreading the infection; and (4) possible spread of infection to involve the joint, causing infectious arthritis, and possible damage to the joint and epiphyseal plate.
4. (pp. 183-184) Anorexia nervosa is extreme weight loss due to self-starvation; bulimia is characterized by binge eating and purging.
5. (p. 185) Epstein-Barr virus (EBV)
6. (p. 185) Manifestations include sore throat, headache, fever, malaise, and fatigue; lymphadenopathy; rash on the trunk; lymphocytosis and monocytosis; and positive heterophil antibody. Complications include hepatitis, ruptured spleen, and meningitis.

CHAPTER 9

Pregnancy

1. (pp. 190-194)
   a) milk production; vi. lactation
   b) premature separation of the placenta from the uterine wall; v. abruptio placentae
   c) pregnancy; i. gestation
   d) inflammation of uterine lining; vii. endometritis
   e) severe hypertension which occurs as a complication of pregnancy; iv. eclampsia
   f) number of pregnancies; ii. gravidity
   g) number of viable pregnancies; iii. parity
2. (pp. 194-197)
   ectopic pregnancy—tubal pregnancy, when the fertilized ovum implants outside the uterus
   preeclampsia and eclampsia—pregnancy-induced hypertension
   gestational diabetes mellitus—increased glucose intolerance and blood glucose levels
   placental problems:
   placenta previa—when the placenta is implanted in the lower uterus or over the os
   abruptio placentae—premature separation of the placenta
   blood clotting problems:
   thrombophlebitis and thromboembolism—clot formation in the veins of the legs or pelvis and potential for embolization if clot breaks free
   disseminated intravascular coagulation
   Rh incompatibility—immune response of Rh negative mother to Rh positive fetal antigens, resulting in anti-Rh antibodies in the maternal bloodstream; i.e., maternal anti-Rh sensitization with potential

for haemolytic disease during subsequent pregnancies.
   infection
   adolescent pregnancy
3. (p. 195 and Fig. 9-2, p. 196) Rh-negative mother exposed to Rh-positive blood via transfusion or pregnancy with Rh-positive fetus; immune response, anti-Rh sensitization resulting in potential for haemolytic disease in subsequent Rh-positive pregnancies
4. (p. 195) Rh immunoglobulin, containing anti-Rh antibodies; when given to an Rh-negative woman who has not been previously sensitized, confers temporary passive immunity and thus prevents maternal sensitization to Rh antigen.

CHAPTER 10

Aging

1. (pp. 202-208)
   i. endocrine system: In general, hormone secretions remain the same, but tissue receptor sensitivity diminishes (see reproductive system for additional female changes; i.e., menopause).
   ii. reproductive system: male: gradual decline in testosterone, decrease in testes size and sperm production but remain potent or fertile; female: menopause, when ovaries cease production of estrogen and progesterone, resulting in rise in serum levels of FSH and LH; decreased sex hormone levels result in thinning of the mucosa, loss of elasticity and glandular secretions in the vagina and cervix which may cause inflammation and dyspareunia; pH of vaginal secretions become more alkaline, predisposing to infections; breasts decrease in size; "hot flashes" due to hormone level changes; signs and symptoms of PMS
   iii. cardiovascular system: fatty tissue and collagen fibers accumulate in heart muscle; size and number of cardiac muscle cells decline; reducing strength of cardiac contractions. Vascular degeneration reduces cardiac output and reserve. Degenerative changes promote arteriosclerosis and atherosclerosis.
   iv. musculoskeletal system: osteoporosis, osteoarthritis, degeneration of intervertebral discs increase risk of herniation or rupture, atrophy of skeletal muscle
   v. respiratory system: ventilation decreases due to reduction in lung tissue elasticity; calcification of costal cartilage reduces movement; skeletal muscle atrophy; vascular degeneration leads to decreased perfusion and gas exchange
   vi. nervous system: various degenerative changes in the brain; decline in various functions, including reflexes, memory, etc.; diminished ANS adaptability; leading to temperature

sensitivities; degenerative changes in the eye resulting in various conditions such as presbyopia, cataracts; glaucoma; hearing loss; diminished sense of taste and smell—appetite loss

    vii. gastrointestinal system: increased risk of oral infections, periodontal disease, loss of teeth; decreased appetite, potential malnutrition; diminished salivation causes difficulty chewing and swallowing, xerostomia (dry mouth); swallowing difficulties due to medications or other neurological problems; obesity and associated disease risks: e.g., diabetes, gallstones, hypertension; atrophy of GI tract mucosa causing malabsorption of essential nutrients, including vitamins and minerals; predisposition to malignancy

    viii. urinary system: reduced kidney function; reduced bladder control

2. (p. 208) Infections are common due to impaired circulation and delayed or diminished healing capacity; diminished immune responsivity; urinary system disorders requiring frequent catheterization, predisposing to infection. Cancer risk is higher due to diminished immune system capabilities and life-long exposure to carcinogens.

3. (pp. 202-209)
   a) inability to control urination; v. incontinence
   b) farsightedness; vii. presbyopia
   c) predetermined cell death; iii. apoptosis
   d) elasticity of the lungs; ix. compliance
   e) excessive urination at night; vi. nocturia
   f) opacity of the ocular lens; ii. cataract
   g) deposition of fat in arterial walls; i. atherosclerosis
   h) dry mouth; viii. xerostomia
   i) increased intraocular pressure; iv. glaucoma

CHAPTER 11

Effects of Immobility

1. (pp. 212-215)
   musculoskeletal effects: muscles lose strength, endurance and mass very quickly atrophy and develop flaccidity; impaired venous return, development of dependent edema; bone demineralization leading to osteoporosis

   cutaneous effects: impaired circulation leads to skin breakdown and reduced regeneration; decubitus ulcers

   circulatory effects: reduced venous return and cardiac output; orthostatic hypotension; blood pooling in dependent areas, resulting in edema; thrombus formation; potential embolism

   respiratory effects: decreased depth of respirations; diminished gaseous exchange; diminished cough resulting in fluid, secretion accumulation; predisposition to respiratory complications: infection, obstruction, and atelectasis; potential for food and water aspiration

gastrointestinal effects: constipation; appetite reduction: malnutrition, fatigue, and depression

urinary effects: urinary stasis with potential for calculus formation and UTI

effects on children: normal growth delayed; spinal or bony deformities; other developmental disorders

2. (pp. 212-214)
   a) stationary blood clot; viii. thrombus
   b) collapse of lung tissue; i. atelectasis
   c) sudden drop in blood pressure when change in position; vi. orthostatic hypotension
   d) floating blood clot; iv. embolus
   e) pressure sore or bedsore; iii. decubitus ulcer
   f) paralysis below the waist; vii. paraplegia
   g) joint deformity caused by excessive scarring; ii. contracture
   h) paralysis of one side of the body; v. hemiplegia

CHAPTER 12

The Influence of Stress

1. (Fig. 12-1, p. 219) Norepinephrine from the SNS and from the adrenal medulla causes general vasoconstriction and increased blood pressure

   Epinephrine from the adrenal medulla causes increased heart rate and general vasoconstriction, resulting in increased blood pressure, vasodilation in skeletal muscle, bronchodilation, and increased blood glucose

   ACTH from the anterior pituitary stimulates the adrenal cortex

   Cortisol from the adrenal cortex results in increased stability in the cardiovascular system and enhances the effects of the catecholamines, elevates blood glucose, reduces the inflammatory and immune responses, and stimulates the CNS

   Aldosterone from the adrenal cortex increases the reabsorption of sodium and water, increasing blood pressure

   ADH from the posterior pituitary increases retention of water, increasing blood pressure

2. (pp. 219-220, Fig. 12-1, p. 219) Significant effects of the sympathetic nervous system during the stress response include elevated blood pressure and increased heart rate, bronchodilation and increased ventilation, increased blood glucose levels, and CNS arousal.

3. (pp. 220-222) Prolonged stress can lead to a variety of serious complications, including disruption of intellectual function and memory, renal failure or stress ulcers. Severe stress can also lead to infection due to depression of the inflammatory response and the immune system. Opportunistic infections may develop, and normally nonpathogenic organisms may cause infection. Continued stress may impede the healing of tissue following trauma or surgery. This may lead to increased risks for infection and scar tissue at the site.

CHAPTER 13

Pain

1. (p. 226) inflammation; infection; ischemia and tissue necrosis; stretching of tissue; chemicals; burns
2. (Fig. 13-1, p. 227, pp. 226-228)
   - stimulation of pain receptors (nociceptors) by thermal, chemical, or physical stimuli
   - if the stimulus exceeds the *threshold* of the receptors, the associated nerve fibers transmit "pain" signal to the spinal cord and brain.
   - myelinated A delta fibers (acute pain) or unmyelinated C fibers (chronic pain) transmit the afferent pain impulse to the dorsal root ganglia and then to the spinal cord.
   - sensory impulse reaches the spinal cord synapse and from there crosses over to the opposite spinothalamic tract (neospinothalamic tract for acute sharp pain; paleospinothalamic tract for chronic or dull pain). [Reflex response to sudden pain at the spinal cord level results in involuntary muscle contraction to move the body part away from the source of pain.]
   - the impulse moves up the lateral spinothalamic tract to the reticular formation (influencing brain awareness) in the brainstem, the hypothalamus (stress response), the thalamus, and other structures (limbic system; emotional response) as they ascend to the
   - somatic sensory area of the cerebral cortex and the parietal lobe of the brain, where the location and character of the pain are perceived.

3. (p. 230, Fig. 13-3, p. 231) Referred pain occurs when pain is perceived at a site distant from the source. It occurs due to multiple sensory fibers from different sources connecting at a single level of the spinal cord, making it difficult for the brain to discern the actual origin of the pain. An example is the pain of a heart attack, which is experienced in the left neck and/or arm.

4. (pp. 234-236, Tables 13-2, 13-3) Pain can be managed in a number of ways. The most common method of management is use of analgesic medications to relieve pain. Sedatives and antianxiety drugs are often used to promote rest and relaxation. Using them in conjunction with analgesics may reduce the dosage of pain medication required. Severe pain may be self-managed by the patient through use of patient-controlled analgesia (PCA). A small pump attached to a vascular access site allows the patient to medicate as needed and reduces the overall amount of narcotic needed. Other methods for managing pain include stress reduction and relaxation, distractors, heat and cold applications, massage, physiotherapy, exercise, therapeutic touch, hypnosis imaging, and acupuncture, which may modify the brain's pain perception and response. Finally, surgical intervention may be necessary to sever the sensory nerve pathway. Injections may be used to achieve similar effects.

5. (p. 232) age, culture, family traditions, and prior experience
6. (Table 13-2, p. 234, pp. 234-235)

	Non-Narcotic Analgesics	Narcotic Analgesics
Action	Decrease pain at peripheral site; all are antipyretic; ASA and NSAIDs are also anti-inflammatory	1. Codeine and oxycodone: act on opiate receptors in the CNS and affect pain perception 2. Morphine and meperidine: act on CNS, producing euphoria and sedation; block pain pathways in the spinal cord and brain
Adverse effects	Nausea, gastric ulcers, bleeding, allergies	1. Nausea, constipation, and, at higher doses, respiratory depression 2. Addiction
Uses	For mild pain, especially when inflammation is present	1. Moderate pain 2. Severe pain
Examples	Tylenol, ibuprofen, naproxen, aspirin	1. Codeine, alone or in combination with acetaminophen); oxycodone 2. Morphine; meperidine

7. (pp. 235-236, Table 13-3)
   local: lidocaine, blocks nerve conduction; removal of skin lesion, tooth extraction
   general: intravenous (thiopental) or inhalation (nitrous oxide); loss of consciousness; general surgery

   spinal anesthesia: local anesthetic into sub-arachnoid or epidural space; blocks nerve conduction (sensation) below the level of injection; labor and delivery

170

CHAPTER 14

Substance Abuse

1. (pp. 240-241) central nervous system depressants or tranquilizers; narcotics; stimulants; psychedelics or hallucinogens
2. (pp. 243-244) Complications of substance abuse include overdose—some drugs have very narrow safety range and an increased dose can have toxic effects and cause death; withdrawal—signs and symptoms of the systemic effect of discontinuing a drug on which the body has become dependent may be mild or severe depending on the drug and include irritability, tremors, nausea, vomiting, stomach cramps, hypertension, psychotic episodes, and convulsions; in pregnancy—effects on the fetus of alcohol (fetal alcohol syndrome) or drug abuse include severe congenital defects and newborns with an addiction and problems of withdrawal, e.g., cocaine causes maternal hypertension, decreasing placental blood flow, resulting in developmental defects and premature birth; cardiovascular effects of stimulants cause hypertension and irregular heartbeat with potential for heart attacks, strokes, or heart failure; psychedelic experiences due to hallucinogens may be positive or negative and include acute fear, panic, depression, and increased risk of suicide Physical effects include hypertension, nausea, and tremors, and there may also be memory loss and distortions of perceptions and judgment; infections such as hepatitis B and HIV are common in drug users who share needles; alcohol—alcoholic liver disease or Laënnec's cirrhosis results from chronic alcohol abuse and Wernicke's syndrome and Korsakoff's psychosis.

CHAPTER 15

Environmental Hazards

1. (pp. 248-252)
   - chemicals—e.g., PCBs, DDT
   - heavy metals—e.g., lead, mercury
   - inhalants—e.g., asbestos, silica, sulfur, various volatile solvents
   - hyperthermia—when environmental temperature is very high and exceeds body's capacity to adapt, especially elderly people
   - hypothermia—e.g., frostbite (localized); systemic exposure such as immersion in very cold water, lack of appropriate clothing in severe cold weather
   - radiation—skin cancer from excessive, chronic exposure to UV irradiation; chronic exposure to household radiation (radon gas)
   - noise—gunshot, loud music
   - bites and stings—neurotoxins of poisonous snakes and spiders
   - food poisoning—from contaminated food or water

CHAPTER 16

Introduction to Basic Pharmacology and Selected Therapies

1. (p. 256) to promote healing, cure disease, control or slow progress of a disease, prevent disease, decrease the risk of complications, increase comfort levels, provide replacement therapy, and reduce excessive activity in the body
2. (p. 256) Therapeutic effect is the desired action; adverse (severe) or side (mild) effects are the unwanted or undesirable effects.
3. (p. 258 and Table 16-1, p. 259)
   i. applied to the skin or mucous membranes; e.g., steroid cream, local anesthetics, antimicrobials, eye drops
   ii. patch applied to the skin for absorption into the blood; e.g., long-term continuous administration of nitroglycerin, nicotine patch, scopolamine patch, estradiol
   iii. by mouth; e.g., aspirin, vitamins, cough syrup, antibiotics
   iv. under the tongue; e.g., nitroglycerin, loperamide, testosterone
   v. injection beneath the epidermis and dermis, into the subcutaneous layer of the skin; e.g., insulin, heparin, interferon
   vi. injection into the muscle; e.g., penicillin, meperidine, tetanus and diphtheria toxoid, vitamin B_{12}
   vii. injection into a vein, into the bloodstream; e.g., general anesthetic like sodium pentothal, morphine, diazepam, vincristine
   viii. into the respiratory tract; e.g., bronchodilator medication, glucocorticoid inhaler, anesthetics such as nitrous oxide
4. (Table 16-1, p. 259) topical
5. (Table 16-1, p. 259)

	Onset of Action	Advantages	Disadvantages
Topical	Rapid	Easy to apply	Can be messy or difficult to apply
Transdermal	Rapid; long term, continuous	Easy to apply for long-term, continuous administration	Action continues after desired effect achieved
Oral	Long time to onset (30-60 min)	Tablets, capsules, stable, variable but relatively inexpensive; self-administered	Taste and swallowing problems; gastric irritation; uncertain absorption
Sublingual	Immediate	Rapid and prolonged effect; can be administered to unconscious patient	Tablets are soft and unstable
Subcutaneous	Slow absorption; some drug loss	Simplest injection; only small doses may be given	Requires asepsis and equipment; may be irritating
Intramuscular	Good absorption into blood, sometimes lag and drug loss	Rapid, prolonged effect; can be used when patient unconscious or nauseated	Requires asepsis and equipment; short shelf-life; some injection discomfort
Intravenous	Immediate and no drug loss	Immediate effect; predictable drug levels; can be used when patient unconscious	Costly; injection skill required; no recovery if drug irritation at the site
Inhalation	Rapid; little loss of drug	Local effect or absorb into alveolar capillaries; rapid; good for anesthesia	Requires effective technique

6. (Table 16-1, p. 259)
   intravenous
   sublingual
   inhalation and topical
   subcutaneous
   intramuscular
   oral

7. (pp. 260-261, Fig. 16-2) Once in the bloodstream, the circulating blood transports drugs via various pathways, branching off into different organs or tissues. Depending on the specific characteristics of a drug, some may be lost temporarily in storage areas such as fatty tissue (e.g., anesthetics) or may be quickly metabolized. Eventually, the drug reaches the target organ or tissue, moves into the interstitial fluid, and exerts its effect. Most drugs are gradually metabolized and inactivated in the liver and then excreted in the kidneys—a few in the bile or feces.

8. (p. 261, Fig. 16-3) Drugs interact with natural specific tissue receptors and act by either (a) stimulating the receptors, increasing biological activity; or (b) blocking the receptor sites, decreasing activity.

9. (p. 261) Drugs are removed from the circulation in the liver, where they are absorbed by the cells whose various metabolic pathways catabolize them.

10. (p. 26) by the kidneys

11. (Think About) Disease of the liver could impair or slow drug metabolism; therefore, the drug is active longer. This prolongs the drug's effects. If the individual is taking the drug regularly, blood levels would gradually increase, possibly resulting in toxic effects. Liver disease may result in decreased production of plasma proteins. This results in decreased protein-binding, resulting in increased free drug in circulation and therefore increased drug effects. Kidney disease may interfere with drug excretion—the drug and its metabolites could accumulate, resulting in increased and prolonged drug effects.

12. (Think About) Inhalation anesthetics are generally excreted via the lungs; it would be difficult to predict the individual's response. There would be problems assessing both the dosage and the rate of drug removal. Intravenous anesthetics depress the respiratory center. This could cause additional hypoxia and increase the risk of developing acidosis.

13. (Think About)
   i. age:
      newborns and babies: immature liver and drug effects more difficult to predict; also have much smaller body mass
      elderly: may have diseases that interfere with drug metabolism and excretion; also more likely to be taking more than one medication, increasing the possibility of drug interactions
   ii. body weight: smaller individuals require less medication—for children, generally dosage calculated according to body weight (p. 257)
   iii. sex:
      Pregnant women should avoid drug usage whenever possible because many drugs cross the placenta and may cause teratogenic effects. (p. 257)

Breastfeeding women should also avoid drug use because many drugs are excreted to some degree in milk and could exert effects on the child.

Gender differences—metabolism, percent body fat, percent body fluids

   iv. psychological factors/emotional state:

If an individual believes a drug is going to be effective, this will likely have a positive effect; the converse is true.

positive suggestion or reinforcement therefore often useful

"placebo" effect (p. 263)

   v. presence of disease (e.g., heart disease; liver disease; kidney disease; etc.):

Heart disease may impair circulation, resulting in decreased distribution, metabolism, and excretion of drugs.

Disease of the liver could impair or slow drug metabolism. Therefore, the drug is active longer—this prolongs the drug's effects. If the individual is taking the drug regularly, blood levels would gradually increase, possibly resulting in toxic effects.

Liver disease may result in decreased production of plasma proteins. This results in decreased protein-binding, resulting in increased free drug in circulation and therefore increased drug effects.

Kidney disease may interfere with drug excretion. Therefore the drug and its metabolites could accumulate, resulting in increased and prolonged drug effects.

   vi. time of administration (in relation to meals; what time of day): (pp. 257-258)

Some medications should be taken with food, while others must be taken on an empty stomach to prevent food interactions. It is therefore important to always confirm with pharmacist, nurse, or physician.

Certain drugs should not be taken at bedtime, e.g., diuretics (water pills, stimulants).

Antibiotics should be evenly spaced throughout the day.

   vii. route of administration: (pp. 259-260, Table 16-1)

determines onset of action

also determines whether there may be drug destruction, e.g., oral route—drug may be destroyed by gastric pH or by food

   viii. drug dosage: (p. 257-258) Generally, the higher the dosage, the greater is the therapeutic effect. Unfortunately, as dosage increases, so do the incidence and severity of adverse and even toxic effects.

   ix. drug formulation (i.e., liquid, capsule, enteric coated): (Table 16-1, p. 259) This will determine onset and duration of action (e.g., liquids absorbed faster than pills; enteric coating will delay onset and may prolong duration of action).

   x. client compliance (i.e., individual's adherence to instructions): (p. 260) Is client taking the drug at prescribed times, with or without food?

   xi. environmental factors (temperature, odors, noise):

Quiet, stress-free environment will enhance effectiveness of analgesics by helping the individual relax.

If someone has just vomited, removal of emesis and opening window to improve ventilation will enhance effectiveness of antiemetic.

   xii. drug interactions: (p. 257)

These may enhance or decrease drug action; e.g., ingestion of alcohol will potentiate narcotics, hypnotics, and sedatives, and caffeine will antagonize hypnotics and sedatives.

14. (pp. 257; 263)
   i. allergic, immunological reaction; e.g. penicillin allergy
   ii. unexpected or unusual responses to drugs; e.g., excessive excitement after administration of a sedative
   iii. where one drug enhances the action of another; e.g., epinephrine enhances the effects of local anesthetic, without increasing the dose
   iv. the effect of a combination of drugs is much greater than expected; e.g., combination of drugs to treat pain
   v. the effects of a combination of drugs is greatly decreased; e.g., antidotes for poisoning
   vi. drugs that produce harmful effects on the fetus during gestation; e.g., narcotics, alcohol
   vii. when the body adapts to a drug, over time, resulting in a higher dosage to achieve the desired effect (See also Chapter 14, Substance Abuse, p. 240.)
   viii. therapeutic effects after administration of a substance that does not have the pharmacologic effects of the drug being studied. (p. 263)

15. (p. 262) Generic names are unique, official, simple names for specific drugs; chemical names reflect the often complex chemical structure of the drug.

16. (pp. 263-267)
   i. individualized treatment and rehabilitation to restore function as well as reduce pain, involving various modalities including exercises, ultrasound, and TENS
   ii. assessment and treatment of communication or swallowing disorders
   iii. functional assessment and treatments to restore activities of daily living (ADLs)
   iv. use of plant, animal, and mineral products to stimulate the immune system and natural healing power of the body
   v. medical practice using surgery and drugs in addition to manipulations of the musculoskeletal system to promote healing
   vi. use of essential oils from plants that have therapeutic effects when applied topically or inhaled

CHAPTER 17

Blood and Lymphatic Disorders

1. (Fig. 17-2, p. 274, pp. 273-274, Fig. 17-4, p. 275) All blood cells originate in the red bone marrow from pluripotential hematopoietic stem cells during hemopoiesis. The life span is approximately 120 days. As the cell ages, it becomes rigid and fragile and finally is phagocytosed in the spleen or liver and broken down into globin and heme. Globin is broken down into amino acids and, along with the iron, is recycled to the liver to be used in hemoglobin synthesis. The heme is processed to release iron for recycling, and bilirubin, which is transported to the liver, where it is conjugated with glucuronide and then excreted in the bile.

2. Handy tables (front cover)
   males:

   RBC: $4.9–5.9 \times 10^6/mm^3$ ($4.9–5.9 \times 10^{12}/L$)

   hemoglobin: 13.5–18 g/100 ml (135–180 g/L)

   females:

   RBC: $4.2–5.2 \times 10^6/mm^3$ ($4.2–5.2 \times 10^{12}/L$)

   hemoglobin: 12–16 g/100 ml (120–160 g/L)

3. (p. 280) below normal concentrations of red blood cells and hemoglobin in the blood
4. (p. 280) fatigue, pallor, dyspnea, and tachycardia
5. (Table 17-2, p. 289)

Type of Anemia	Etiology	Specific Manifestations	Specific Treatment
Iron deficiency anemia (pp. 280-282, Fig. 17-9, p. 281)	Malnutrition Chronic blood loss Malabsorption Severe liver disease Under utilization of iron in some infections and cancers	Pallor Fatigue, lethargy, and cold intolerance Irritability Degenerative changes: e.g., brittle hair, rigid nails Stomatitis and glossitis Menstrual irregularities Delayed healing Tachycardia, heart palpitations, dyspnea, and possible syncope	Identify and treat the underlying cause Iron supplements
Pernicious anemia— vitamin B_{12} deficiency anemia (pp. 282-284, Fig. 17-10, p. 283)	Dietary insufficiency (rare) Malabsorption resulting from autoimmune reaction; chronic gastritis; or inflammatory conditions (e.g., regional ileitis)	Basic signs of anemia Enlarged, red, sore tongue Decreased gastric acid leading to discomfort, nausea, and diarrhea Neurological effects: paresthesia in the extremities or loss of coordination and ataxia	Vitamin B_{12} replacement therapy; vitamin B_{12} injection
Aplastic anemia (pp. 284-285)	(Temporary or permanent) Idiopathic Myelotoxins (e.g., radiation, industrial chemicals, certain drugs)	Anemia (pallor, weakness, dyspnea) Leukopenia Thrombocytopenia (petechiae; excessive bleeding)	Prompt treatment of the underlying cause and removal of any bone marrow suppressants Blood transfusion Bone marrow transplant
Thalassemia (pp. 288-289)	Genetic defect in which one or more genes for hemoglobin are missing or variant	Anemia (pallor, weakness, dyspnea)	Blood transfusion

Type of Anemia, cont'd	Etiology, cont'd	Specific Manifestations, cont'd	Specific Treatment, cont'd
Sickle cell anemia (pp. 285-288, Figs. 17-12, 17-13, 17-14)	Inherited characteristic leading to the formation of an abnormal hemoglobin (HbS)	(Usually appears at about 1 year of age when fetal hemoglobin is replaced by HbS) Severe anemia (pallor, weakness, tachycardia, and dyspnea) Hyperbilirubinemia (jaundice) Splenomegaly Painful crises due to vascular occlusion and infarction Delayed growth and development Congestive heart failure Frequent infections	Drugs that reduce sickling, e.g., hydroxyurea Avoidance of strenuous activity or high altitudes Supportive measures

6. See Figure 17-14 (p. 287) for pattern of inheritance. Inheritance pattern is autosomal recessive; the genotype of an individual with sickle cell anemia is homozygous.

7. (p. 286) The individual is heterozygous for sickle cell anemia. Less than half of his hemoglobin is abnormal; therefore, he experiences manifestations only in extreme circumstances.

8. (p. 287)

	Mother with Sickle Cell Trait	
Father with Sickle Cell Anemia	s	a
s	ss anemia	sa trait
s	ss anemia	sa trait

i. Probability that the child will have sickle cell anemia? 50%

ii. Probability that the child will have sickle cell trait? 50%

iii. Probability that the child will have neither sickle cell trait nor disease? 0%

iv. Probability that any future child whom this couple conceives will have sickle cell anemia? 50%

9. (pp. 285-286, Fig. 17-13, p. 287) An inherited, abnormal form of hemoglobin (HbS) is circulating in the bloodstream. When these RBCs are deoxygenated, they crystalize and change shape. The cell membrane is damaged, leading to hemolysis and shorter cell life span. The sickled cells cause vascular obstruction, thrombus formation, tissue infarction, and necrosis. Continued hemolysis results in severe anemia, hyperbilirubinemia, jaundice, splenomegaly, and gallstones.

10. (p. 285, Figs. 17-12 and 17-13, pp. 286-287) deoxygenation of abnormal hemoglobin when O_2 levels are low

11. (p. 287) periodic painful episodes due to vascular occlusions and infarctions leading to permanent damage to organs and tissues; potential complications such as infection and congestive heart failure

12. (pp. 285-288, Fig. 17-13, p. 287)
   i. jaundice: excessive hemolysis, RBC breakdown, and resulting hyperbilirubinemia
   ii. cerebrovascular accident: cerebrovascular occlusion by sickled cells
   iii. frequent infections: diminished immune capacity (damage to spleen); vascular occlusions in the lungs; tissue damage and necrosis
   iv. splenomegaly: congestion of the spleen due to presence of sickled cells in young people
   v. congestive heart failure: chronic stress on the heart due to efforts to improve oxygen supply and peripheral vascular resistance due to obstructions

13. (p. 288) genetic screening to identify carriers and genetic counselling to discern the risks of having a child with sickle cell anemia

14. (p. 289) Polycythemia is increased red blood cell and other cell production in the bone marrow.

15. (p. 289) Primary polycythemia is a neoplastic disorder of unknown origin, whereas secondary polycythemia may be a compensatory mechanism to provide increased oxygen transport in the presence of lung or heart disease or in people living at high altitudes.

16. (p. 289) manifestations: plethoric and cyanotic appearance; hepatomegaly; high blood pressure; full and bounding pulse; dyspnea, headaches, and visual disturbances

complications: thromboses and infarctions in extremities, liver, kidneys, brain and heart; congestive heart failure

17. (p. 290) immunosuppressive drugs, radiation, and periodic phlebotomy

18. See Figure 17-6 (p. 276) of the main text.

19. (Warning Signs of Excessive Bleeding box, p. 290)

persistent bleeding from the gums or frequent nosebleeds

petechiae

frequent purpura and ecchymoses

abnormal persistent bleeding following trauma

bleeding into a joint

hemoptysis

hematemesis—vomiting blood

blood in the feces

anemia

feeling faint and anxious, low blood pressure, rapid pulse

20. (p. 278) CBC; hematocrit; hemoglobin; reticulocyte count; bone marrow aspiration and biopsy; serum iron, vitamin B_{12}, folic acid, cholesterol, urea, and bilirubin; bleeding time; prothrombin time; partial thromboplastin time

21. (pp. 290-291, Fig. 17-6, p. 276)

thrombocytopenia (many causes; e.g., autoimmune reactions): reduced circulating platelets that initiate the clotting process

defective platelet adhesion caused by ASA and NSAIDs

vitamin K deficiency: decreases prothrombin and fibrinogen levels

liver disease: interferes with the production of clotting factors

inherited defects: cause deficiency in clotting factors

anticoagulant drugs: e.g., warfarins block prothrombin synthesis

22. (pp. 290-291, Fig. 17-6, p. 276)

    i. liver disease: delayed clotting—due to decreased synthesis of clotting factors

    ii. ingestion of ASA: delayed clotting—decreased aggregation or clumping of platelet

    iii. prolonged antibiotic therapy: delayed clotting—vitamin K, which is necessary for production of clotting factors, is synthesized by resident flora of large intestine; prolonged antibiotic therapy may disrupt or destroy flora

    iv. administration of heparin: delayed clotting—heparin inhibits thrombin formation

    v. vitamin K deficiency: delayed clotting—vitamin K necessary for synthesis of clotting factors by liver

    vi. prolonged inactivity (e.g., postoperatively or sitting on a airplane for many hours): promotes clotting—decreased blood velocity, resulting in pooling of blood

    vii. polycythemia: promotes clotting—increased blood viscosity, which decreases blood velocity and promotes pooling

    viii. thrombocytopenia: delayed clotting—decreased platelets slow formation of platelet plug

    ix. increased hematocrit: promotes clotting—increased blood viscosity with resultant decreased blood velocity

    x. administration of warfarin (Coumadin): delayed clotting—anticoagulant that decreases synthesis of various clotting factors, particularly prothrombin

23. (p. 291, Fig. 17-16) Hemophilia A is transmitted as an X-linked recessive trait and therefore it manifests in men but women are carriers. Males are heterozygous; females are homozygous.

24. (p. 291)

	Female Carrier	
Father	X	X_h
X	XX normal female	$X\,X_h$ (25%)
Y	XY normal male	$X_h Y$ (25%)

    i. 25%—male

    ii. 25%—female

    iii. 50%

    iv. 50%

    v. 50%

25. (p. 291, Fig. 17-16B)

    i. heterozygous

    ii. heterozygous

(Fig. 17-16B)

    iii. 50%

    iv. 25%

    v. female

26. (p. 292, Fig. 17-17, p. 293) DIC involves excessive bleeding and clotting. It is a complication of numerous primary problems that activates the clotting process. Clotting causes multiple thromboses and infarctions but also consumes the available clotting factors and platelets. This can lead to hemorrhage and eventually hypotension or shock. Manifestations depend on the underlying cause. Hemorrhage is the most common critical problem combined with low blood pressure and possibly shock. Multiple bleeding sites are common, petechiae or ecchymoses may be present, mucosal bleeding is common, and hematuria may develop. Vascular occlusions may be present in the blood vessels. Difficulty in breathing and cyanosis are evident. Neurological effects include seizures and decreased responsiveness. Acute renal failure may accompany shock.

27. (p. 293) Leukemia is a neoplastic disorder involving one or more types of leukocytes that are present as undifferentiated, immature, nonfunctional cells that multiply uncontrollably and are found circulating in large numbers in the blood.

28. (p. 294) Blast cells are primitive undifferentiated non-functional stems cells seen in severe forms of acute leukemia.

29. (p. 294, Table 17-3) acute or chronic; specific cell type involved: e.g., acute lymphocytic (ALL); chronic myelogenous (CML), etc.

30. (p. 285) individuals with chromosomal abnormalities, particularly translocations such as Down syndrome; those exposed to radiation and certain chemicals

31. (p. 295) bone marrow biopsy

32. (pp. 294-295, Fig. 17-19)

Manifestation	Rationale
Weight loss and fatigue	Hypermetabolism associated with neoplastic growth, anorexia due to infection; pain; side effects of chemotherapy
Anemia	Due to hemorrhage and suppression of normal RBC production in the bone marrow
Thrombocytopenia	Suppression of platelet production in the bone marrow by proliferating neoplastic cells
Multiple infections, including those caused by microorganisms of low virulence	Nonfunctional WBCs being produced; diminished primary and secondary defense against infection
Increased bleeding and even severe hemorrhage	Thrombocytopenia
Kidney stones	Rapid turnover of cells leading to hyperuricemia
Fever	Hypermetabolism and/or infection
Lymphadenopathy	Excess production of abnormal leukocytes causes enlargement and congestion of lymphoid tissue
Splenomegaly and hepatomegaly	Excess production of abnormal leukocytes causes enlargement and congestion
Bone pain	Excessive cell production in the marrow causes pain due to pressure on nerves

33. (pp. 295-296, see also Chapter 5) Chemotherapy, singly or in combinations, is the primary treatment. Adverse effects include bone marrow depression, nausea and vomiting, hair loss, and skin breakdown; some drugs cause pulmonary fibrosis. If ineffective, bone marrow transplantation is another intervention. Biologic agents such as interferon to stimulate the immune system may also be used.

34. (pp. 295-296) The best prognosis is in ALL in children between 1 and 9 years of age; less so in adolescents. The prognosis is poor in adults, especially those with AML. Chronic leukemia patients may live up to 10 years. Prognosis depends on WBC and blast counts at diagnosis.

35. (p. 296)

	Acute Leukemia	Chronic Leukemia
Age of onset	Childhood and young adults	Older individuals
Course of disease	Acute onset; rapid development of manifestations	Insidious onset, milder, slower progression
Severity of symptoms	Acute	Milder
Number of blast cells	High	Fewer
Response to treatment	Good in some types	Depends on general health
Prognosis	Excellent in some types	Poorer but over long period of time

36. (p. 296, Fig. 17-20, p. 297) Giant Reed-Sternberg cell is used for diagnosis. It is characterized as a giant irregular cell present in the lymph node.

37. (p. 296, Fig. 17-21, p. 298)
    stage I—single lymph node or region
    stage II—multiple regions on same side of diaphragm
    stage III—lymph node regions on both sides of diaphragm
    stage IV—widespread; liver and spleen

38. (p. 297)
large, painless, nontender lymph node, usually in the neck; splenomegaly and enlarged lymph nodes at other locations later; general signs of cancer such as weight loss, anemia, low-grade fever, night sweats, and fatigue; recurrent infection

39. (p. 297) radiation, chemotherapy (especially ABVD combo), and surgery

40. (p. 297) Non-Hodgkin's lymphoma is distinguished by multiple node involvement scattered throughout the body in nonorganized pattern of widespread metastasis; intestinal nodes are frequently involved in the early stages.

41. (p. 297) a neoplastic disease of unknown etiology involving plasma cells

42. (pp. 297-298) Manifestations include frequent infections due to impaired antibody production; bone pain due to production of excess plasma cells in the marrow; pathological fractures due to the weakened bones; anemia and bleeding tendencies because blood cell production is compromised; and proteinuria due to altered kidney function.

43. (p. 272)
   i. diagnosed by presence of Reed-Sternberg cells: Hodgkin's
   ii. involves both excessive bleeding and clotting: disseminated intravascular coagulation
   iii. decreased or lack of intrinsic factor production: pernicious anemia
   iv. characterized by primitive blast cells: leukemia (especially acute)
   v. sex-linked bleeding disorder: hemophilia A
   vi. increased production of erythrocytes: polycythemia
   vii. frequent adverse effect of chemotherapy: aplastic anemia, leukopenia, thrombocytopenia
   viii. may result in impaired growth and development: sickle cell anemia
   ix. common in individuals from the Mediterranean area: thalassemia
   x. may be accompanied by jaundice: sickle cell anemia
   xi. may be accompanied by loss of coordination: pernicious anemia, vitamin B_{12} deficiency anemia
   xii. a neoplastic disorder involving the red blood cells: polycythemia vera
   xiii. more prevalent in individuals with Down syndrome: leukemia
   xiv. generalized pruritis is common: Hodgkin's
   xv. predisposes individual to infections: leukemia, anemia (especially aplastic and sickle cell), Hodgkin's, multiple myeloma

CHAPTER 18

Cardiovascular Disorders

1. (pp. 320-321)
   age—cannot be changed
   gender—cannot be changed
   genetic or familial factors—cannot be changed
   obesity—modifiable
   cigarette smoking—modifiable
   sedentary lifestyle—modifiable
   diabetes mellitus—modifiable
   poorly controlled hypertension—modifiable
   oral contraceptives and smoking in combination—modifiable
   high cholesterol and hypertension—modifiable

2. (pp. 318-319, Fig. 18-12)
   endothelial injury in the artery, often at a young age
   inflammation and elevation of C-reactive protein
   accumulation of white blood cells, especially monocytes and macrophages
   lipid accumulates in the intima or inner lining of the artery and media or muscle layer
   a plaque forms and inflammation persists
   platelets adhere to damaged surface, forming a thrombus and partial obstruction
   continued lipid buildup at the site of injury along with fibrous tissue (atheroma)
   platelets adhere, prostaglandins released, causing further inflammation and vasospasm
   process continues with larger thrombus formation, and potential total occlusion and possibility of embolism

3. (pp. 318-319, Figs. 18-12 and 18-13, p. 321)
   Development of atheromatous plaques narrows the lumen of arteries, restricting flow, causing turbulence, thrombus formation, and potential embolism. The atheroma also damages the arterial wall, weakening the structure and decreasing elasticity, and ultimately may calcify, causing further rigidity. Complications include thrombus formation, with partial (angina) or total occlusion, precipitating a myocardial infarction, embolism and infarction (stroke and peripheral vascular damage), aneurysm, or rupture and hemorrhage.

4. (p. 318) primarily large arteries particularly at bifurcations—aorta, coronary, iliac, carotids

5. (pp. 321-322)
   i. diet: lowering serum cholesterol and LDL by reducing the intake of saturated fats and using unsaturated or vegetable oils; high dietary fiber intake also decreases LDL; sodium intake should be minimized to help control hypertension; weight loss helps control diabetes as well as hypertension
   ii. exercise: reduces blood pressure and stress level and increases HDL while lowering LDL and cholesterol
   iii. medications (Table 18-1, p. 317)
      a. antilipidemics or lipid-lowering drugs: lower cholesterol and LDL levels
      b. platelet inhibitors: lower platelet aggregation leading to a lower chance of thrombosis and thus leading to a lower chance of heart attacks and strokes
      c. anticoagulants: interfere with clotting factor synthesis (warfarin) or inhibit thrombin formation (heparin), leading to a lower chance

of thrombosis and a lower chance of heart attacks and strokes

d. antihypertensives: help decrease cardiac workload

   iv. lifestyle/behavioral modifications: (p. 322) stop smoking, adopt a diet low in saturated and trans fats, restricted sodium intake, weight loss if overweight, consistent exercise program, stress reduction

   v. surgical intervention:

   a. endarterectomy: surgical removal of the intima and obstructive material (p. 348)

   b. angioplasty: various surgical techniques to recanalize or reopen an artery; e.g., PTCA, which involves catherization and flattening of the atheroma by inflation of a balloon attached to the catheter (p. 322)

   c. coronary artery bypass grafting: using veins as vessel graft to bypass the obstructed artery (Fig. 18-14, p. 323)

6. (Fig. 18-1, p. 304)
7. (p. 322) chest pain
8. (p. 322) when there is decreased blood supply (oxygen) to the heart, due to either arterial obstruction or spasm OR

when there is increased demand for oxygen by the heart OR

when there is a combination of factors

9. (p. 324)
atherosclerosis
arteriosclerosis
vasospasm
myocardial hypertrophy
severe anemias
respiratory disease

10. (p. 324) myocardial infarction
11. (p. 324)
   i. smoking a cigarette or being exposed to second-hand smoke: smoke causes vasoconstriction, leading to increased venous return and heart rate

   ii. going from a warm environment into the cold: vasoconstriction, leading to increased venous return and increased heart rate

   iii. engaging in an argument or other stressful behavior: sympathetic stimulation increases heart rate

   iv. exercise, such as climbing a flight of stairs or rushing to catch a bus: increases heart rate due to increased O_2 demands

12. (p. 324, Fig. 18-15, p. 323) The classic manifestations are recurrent, intermittent brief episodes of substernal chest pain, described as a tightness or pressure that may radiate to the neck or left arm. An anginal attack usually lasts a few seconds or minutes.

13. (p. 324) Vasodilators, which act by reducing systemic resistance, thus decrease the demand for oxygen; some relieve arterial vasospasm.

14. (p. 324) Nitroglycerin, which is administered in a sublingual tablet or spray. This route has almost immediate onset of action with no drug loss.

15. (Emergency Treatment Box, p. 324)
16. (Emergency Treatment Box, p. 324)
   if pain is not relieved with rest and administration of three doses of nitroglycerin spaced 5 minutes apart—i.e., after 15 minutes

   for individual with no history of angina, if pain is unrelieved within 2 minutes

17. (Table 18-1, p. 317)

Drug Group	Action and Effects	Adverse Effects	Example
β-Adrenergic blockers	Blocks β-adrenergic receptors, slowing the heart rate, reducing work of the heart	Dizziness, fatigue	Lopressor
Calcium channel blockers	Vasodilator, blocks calcium channel, reducing cardiac contractility and work	Dizziness, fainting, headache	Adalat
Nitrates (vasodilators) (transdermal or oral form)	Reduces cardiac workload; decreases peripheral resistance by vasodilation	Dizziness; headache	Nitroglycerin

18. (Think About)
antihypertensive to lower blood pressure and cardiac workload
diuretic to help control blood pressure and prevent edema
platelet inhibitor to lower platelet aggregation and the chance of thrombus formation
antihyperlidemic to lower blood cholesterol and LDL levels and hopefully slow or arrest progression of atherosclerosis

19. (p. 322) angioplasty and stent insertion; coronary bypass graft

20. (p. 322)
avoid situations known to precipitates attacks, e.g., stress
stop smoking
consume diet low in saturated and trans fats
restrict sodium intake
weight loss if overweight
consistent exercise program
stress reduction

21. (p. 324)
How long has he had angina?
How frequent are attacks?
When was last one?
What are known precipitating factors?
What is his response to nitroglycerin?
Does he have his nitroglycerin with him?
Has he suffered a heart attack?

22. (p. 324)
stress reduction—explanations and reassurance
short appointments
prophylactic use of nitroglycerin

23. (pp. 324-325) death of cardiac muscle resulting from prolonged ischemia

24. (p. 325) Infarction may develop in three ways:
thrombus buildup to obstruct the artery due to atherosclerosis (most common)
vasospasm in the presence of a partial occlusion
embolization of a thrombus to a smaller artery that is totally obstructed

25. (p. 326) pallor, anxiety, fear, diaphoresis, shortness of breath and tightness in chest, weakness, indigestion or nausea

26. (p. 325) Transmural infarction involves all three layers of heart; and a subendocardial infarction involves the inner one-third to one-half of the wall

27. (p. 325) left ventricle

28. (pp. 324-326, Fig. 18-16) Myocardial infarction occurs when a coronary artery is totally occluded, causing prolonged ischemia and cell death or infarction of myocardium. At the point of obstruction, heart tissue becomes necrotic, and an area of injury, inflammation, and ischemia develops around the necrotic zone. Functions of myocardial contractility and conduction are lost quickly. There is irreversible damage unless blood supply can be restored with the first 20 minutes. Inflammation subsides after 48 hours. The area of necrosis is gradually replaced by fibrous (nonfunctional) tissue. The size of the infarct is determined by location of arterial blockage and presence of collateral circulation.

29. (p. 326) Manifestations include sudden, severe, steady, and crushing substernal chest pain that radiates to the left arm, shoulder, jaw, or neck. Other manifestations may occur even if pain is not present, including pallor, diaphoresis, nausea, dizziness, weakness, dyspnea, anxiety, fear, hypotension, and low-grade fever.

30. (p. 326) Diagnosis is confirmed through ECG changes and serum enzyme and isoenzyme levels.

31. (p. 326, Fig. 18-17) Serum enzymes are intracellular enzymes diffused from necrotic cells into the serum in a typical and predictable pattern that can be measured. Isoenzymes are subgroups of a specific enzyme that are found primarily in one type of tissue. Levels of serum enzymes and isoenzymes can be used to identify the site of the infarction, confirm a myocardial infarction, and also assess size (severity) of infarction.

32. (pp. 326-327) Electrical activity of myocardium will be altered in areas of severe ischemia or necrosis.

33. (p. 326) The following diagnostic tools may also diagnose an MI:
serum levels of myosin and troponin elevated, providing for earlier confirmation
serum electrolytes, especially potassium and sodium, may be abnormal
WBC, CRP, and ESR: leukocytosis with elevated CRP and EST common indicators of acute inflammation
arterial blood gases, especially if signs of shock present
pulmonary arterial pressure: indicator of ventricular function

34. (pp. 326-327) Arrhythmias account for the greatest number of deaths because they impair the efficiency of the heart, resulting in decreased perfusion to vital organs as well as the heart itself leading to shock.

35. (p. 327) Other complications include cardiogenic shock, congestive heart failure, rupture of necrotic heart tissue, and thromboembolism.

36. (p. 327) Treatment includes rest, oxygen therapy, analgesics, anticoagulants, antiarrhythmic drugs, digoxin, specific measure to treat shock if present, and bypass surgery.

37. (pp. 322-327)
Angina usually precipitated by something that increases heart rate; an MI may occur at rest or even while asleep.
Anginal pain is relieved by nitroglycerin and rest; the pain of an MI is not relieved by nitroglycerin and rest.
There is no tissue death (permanent damage) with angina; MI causes cell death.
Cardiac enzymes and isoenzymes are elevated with MI; there are no changes with angina. There are permanent ECG changes with MI; no permanent change with angina.
There is leukocytosis with MI, which is not elevated with angina.
CRP is elevated with MI; it is not elevated with angina.
ESR is elevated with MI but not with angina.
There are elevated serum levels of myosin and troponin with MI.

38. (Fig. 18-18, p. 328)

39. (Fig. 18-18, p. 328) SA node to AV node to AV bundle (bundle of His) to right and left bundle branches to Purkinje fibers
40. (Fig. 18-18, p. 328)
41. (Fig. 18-18, p. 328)
    i. P wave: atrial depolarization and contraction
    ii. QRS complex: ventricular depolarization and contraction
    iii. T wave: ventricular repolarization and relaxation
42. (p. 328) alteration of cardiac rate or rhythm
43. (p. 328) Cardiac arrhythmias may occur due to damage to the heart's conduction system or systemic causes such as electrolyte abnormalities, fever, hypoxia, stress, infection, or drug toxicity.
44. (Table 18-2, p. 330)
    a) heart rate greater than 350 beats per minute; v. fibrillation
    b) extra heartbeat arising in the ventricles; viii. premature ventricular contraction (PVC)
    c) heart rate less than 60 beats per minute; ii. bradycardia
    d) slowing or no transmission of impulses between atria and ventricles; vi. heart block
    e) additional heartbeat originating in atria; vii. premature atrial contraction (PAC)
    f) restoration of normal cardiac rhythm by electrical shock; i. cardioversion
    g) heart rate between 160 and 350 beats per minute; iv. flutter
    h) extra beat originating outside the SA node; iii. ectopic beat
    i) heart rate between 100 and 160 beats per minute; ix. tachycardia
45. (pp. 328-329) It interferes with normal ventricular filling and decreases both period of ventricular diastole and perfusion.
46. (p. 329) It results in decreased cardiac output, which results in decreased perfusion of vital organs.
47. (Table 18-1, pp. 315-317)

Drug Group	Action and Effects	Adverse Effects	Example
β-Adrenergic blockers	Blocks β-adrenergic receptors, slowing the heart rate, prevents SNS stimulation and increased demand on heart	Dizziness, fatigue	Lopressor
Calcium channel blockers	Vasodilator, blocks calcium channel	Dizziness, fainting, headache	Adalat
Digitalis (cardiac glycosides)	Slows conduction through the AV node, increases force of contraction (cardiotonic) to increase efficiency	Nausea, fatigue, headache, weakness	Lanoxin

48. (p. 322, Table 18-1, p. 317)
    antihypertensive to decrease blood pressure and cardiac workload
    diuretic to help control blood pressure and prevent edema
    platelet inhibitor to decrease platelet aggregation and decrease the chance of thrombus formation
    anticoagulant to decrease the chance of thrombus formation
    antihyperlidemic to decrease blood cholesterol and LDL levels and hopefully slow or arrest progression of atherosclerosis
    nitroglycerin
49. (p. 330, Fig. 18-20, p. 321) device that provides electrical stimulation directly to the heart muscle to stimulate heart contraction as needed or for overall control of heart rate
50. (p. 330) Use of electronic equipment (microwaves, dental cavitrons) may interfere with normal functioning of pacemaker.
51. (p. 331) Causes include a problem in the heart itself (e.g., valve defect or MI) or a condition that increases the workload of the heart (e.g., hypertension).
52. (pp. 331-332, Fig. 18-21) SNS stimulation causing vasoconstriction and increased resistance for left ventricle and increased heart rate and force leading to increased work for the heart. Renin secretion stimulated by reduced systemic blood flow, causing activation of angiotensin leading to vasoconstriction, stimulation of aldosterone secretion leading to sodium and water retention, increased blood volume, and increased work load for the heart
53. (pp. 332-333, Fig. 18-22) Backward effects: the chamber and blood vessels behind or "upstream" from the failing ventricle will not empty properly, resulting in the accumulation or congestion of blood and therefore an increased pressure in these areas. Forward effects: there will be decreased output of blood from the failing ventricle into the vessels "in front" of it or "downstream."
54. (Table 18-3, pp. 334-335)

	Right-Sided Heart Failure	Left-Sided Heart Failure
Cause	Infarction of right ventricle, pulmonary valve stenosis, pulmonary disease (cor pulmonale)	Infarction of left ventricle, aortic valve stenosis, hypertension, hyperthyroidism
Backward effects	Dependent edema in feet, hepatomegaly and splenomegaly, ascites, distended neck veins, headache, flushed face	Orthopnea, cough, shortness of breath, paroxysmal nocturnal dyspnea, hemoptysis, rales
Forward effects	Fatigue, weakness, dyspnea, exercise intolerance, cold intolerance	Fatigue, weakness, dyspnea, exercise intolerance, cold intolerance
Manifestations	See above forward and backward effects. Compensations: tachycardia and pallor, secondary polycythemia, daytime oliguria	See above forward and backward effects. Compensations: tachycardia and pallor, secondary polycythemia, daytime oliguria

55. (pp. 334-335)
   i. right-sided heart failure: peripheral edema
   ii. left-sided heart failure: shortness of breath or dyspnea, particularly on exertion
56. (pp. 331-335)
   i. splenomegaly: venous congestion in inferior vena cava and other veins draining abdominal organs
   ii. ascites: venous congestion in inferior vena cava and other veins draining abdominal organs
   iii. orthopnea: due to pulmonary edema—fluid shifts into upper lobes when head lowered, causing dyspnea and anxiety, and more fluid shifts from tissues into blood when recumbent, thus increasing vascular volume and pressure in pulmonary capillaries
   iv. cough: due to fluid congestion in lungs and pulmonary edema
   v. hemoptysis: as congestion increased in pulmonary circulation, red blood cells are pushed out of capillaries into alveoli, causing rusty-colored sputum or blood-specked sputum
   vi. distended neck veins: due to increased congestion and pressure in superior vena cava
   vii. decreased urine output: occurs during day—vas fluid accumulates in dependent regions, there is decreased renal perfusion. Late in disease, oliguria reflects decreased cardiac output and renal failure.
   viii. nocturia: when individual is in supine position, edema in dependent areas is mobilized, resulting in increased cardiac output, renal perfusion, and therefore glomerular filtration rate.
   ix. polycythemia: impaired gas exchange due to pulmonary congestion causes chronic hypoxia that in turn stimulates release of erythropoietin—increased RBC production.
57. (p. 336)
   i. low sodium diet: helps prevent fluid retention

ii. low cholesterol diet: hopefully helps arrest progression of atherosclerosis
   iii. compression stockings: prevent venous stasis and thrombophlebitis
   iv. continuous oxygen therapy: decreases dyspnea and improves arterial blood gases
   v. diuretics: mobilize edema (including pulmonary edema) and promote excretion of excess fluid leading to decreased plasma volume and therefore decreased cardiac workload
   vi. potassium supplement: to prevent hypokalemia, which is a common side effect of diuretic therapy
   vii. angiotensin-converting enzyme (ACE) inhibitors: decrease renin secretion and therefore prevent both vasoconstriction and aldosterone secretion (which causes salt and water retention)
   viii. digoxin: increases strength of myocardial contractions that increase cardiac output
   ix. platelet inhibitor or anticoagulant: decreases thrombosis, particularly in legs
   x. sedative or antianxiety agent: decreases anxiety, which can contribute to increased heart and respiratory rates
58. (p. 337) Most defects are multifactorial and reflect both genetic and environmental influences: e.g., chromosomal abnormalities in Down syndrome. Environmental factors include viral infections such as rubella and maternal alcoholism (FAS) and diabetes.
59. (pp. 338-340, Fig. 18-24, p. 336, Fig. 18-25, p. 337)
   i. septal defect: a hole or defect in the atrial or ventricular septa
   ii. valvular incompetence: failure of a valve to close completely
   iii. regurgitation: backward flow or leaking of blood due to valvular incompetence

iv. prolapse: abnormally enlarged and floppy valve leaflets that balloon backward with pressure or posterior displacement of the valve cusp

v. stenosis: narrowing of a valve

vi. heart murmur: abnormal heart sounds due to leaky valves (p. 308)

60. (p. 338) by presence of a heart murmur

61. (pp. 338-339) lowers O_2 supply to tissues unless adequate compensations available

62. (pp. 337-338) Left-to-right shunt means that blood from the left side of the heart is recycled to the right side and to the lungs, resulting in increased volume in the pulmonary circulation, a decreased cardia output, and an inefficient system—an acyanotic condition. Right-to-left shunt means that unoxygenated blood from the right side of the heart bypasses the lung directly and enters the left side of the heart and hence the systemic circulation, producing varying degrees of cyanosis; death may occur in infancy in severe cases

63. (p. 338) Manifestations include pallor and cyanosis

tachycardia, with very rapid sleeping pulse frequently a pulse deficit

dyspnea on exertion and tachypnea

in toddlers and older children, frequently assuming a squatting position to modify blood flow

children frequently show marked intolerance for exercise and exposure to cold

delayed growth and development

64. (pp. 337-338, Fig. 18-25) Left-to-right shunt, reducing the flow of blood from the left ventricle, reducing stroke volume and cardiac output in the systemic circulation. More blood enters the pulmonary circulation, compromising its efficiency, and in time, overloads and irreversibly damages the pulmonary vessels, causing pulmonary hypertension. This complication, if untreated, would lead to abnormally high pressure in the right ventricle and reversal of the shunt to a right-to-left shunt, leading to cyanosis.

65. (pp. 336-340; Figs. 18-24 to 18-27)

Defect	Backward Effects	Forward Effects	Manifestations
Mitral stenosis	Left atrial hypertrophy Atrial arrhythmias Mural thrombi Pulmonary congestion Pulmonary hypertension	Decreased cardiac output	Dyspnea, orthopnea Cyanosis, fatigue Arrhythmias Heart murmur Increased risk of stroke due to emboli originating in left atrium
Mitral regurgitation	Left atrial hypertrophy Atrial arrhythmias Mural thrombi Pulmonary congestion Pulmonary hypertension	Decreased cardiac output	Dyspnea, orthopnea Cyanosis, fatigue, dizziness Arrhythmias Heart murmur
Aortic stenosis	Left ventricular hypertrophy If severe, increased congestion in left atrium and pulmonary congestion	Decreased cardiac output	Dizziness, fainting Fatigue Heart murmur If severe, dyspnea, orthopnea, cyanosis Angina
Aortic regurgitation	Left ventricular hypertrophy If severe, heart failure	Increased stroke volume and cardiac output	Very strong, bounding pulse Heart murmur May develop symptoms of heart failure

Defect, cont'd	Backward Effects, cont'd	Forward Effects, cont'd	Manifestations, cont'd
Pulmonary stenosis	Right ventricular hypertrophy Congestion in right atrium and systemic veins Leads to right-sided heart failure	Decreased blood flow through pulmonary circulation leading to decreased gas exchange and blood to left side of heart	Weakness, fatigue, cyanosis Swelling of feet and ankles Symptoms of right-sided heart failure Heart murmur
Pulmonary regurgitation	Right ventricular hypertrophy Congestion in right atrium and systemic veins Leads to right-sided heart failure	Decreased blood flow through pulmonary circulation leading to decreased gas exchange and blood to left side of heart	Weakness, fatigue, cyanosis Swelling of feet and ankles Symptoms of right-sided heart failure Heart murmur

66. (pp. 336-338) valvular defect; septal defect
67. (p. 341, Fig. 18-25C, p. 340)
   pulmonary valve stenosis: restricts outflow from the right ventricle, leading to right ventricular hypertrophy and high pressure in the right ventricle leading to the right-to-left shunt
   ventricular septal defect (VSD): an opening in the ventricular septum allows blood to flow between the ventricles
   dextroposition of the aorta: promotes blood flow directly from the right ventricle into the general circulation
   right ventricular hypertrophy: thickening of the ventricular wall because of increased work
   The most common cyanotic congenital heart disorder, tetralogy of Fallot is a right-to-left shunt of blood through the VSD with marked systemic effects. This means that unoxygenated blood from the right side of the heart bypasses the lungs and enters the left side of the heart and into the general circulation. The high proportion of unoxygenated blood produces a bluish color in the skin and mucous membranes (cyanosis) and marked systemic effects resulting from hypoxemia.
68. (p. 338) Interventions include surgical repair of defect, valve replacement, or drug therapy (those used for heart failure).
69. (p. 338)
   i. He will be taking a platelet inhibitor such as ASA or an anticoagulant because despite replacement of damaged valve, platelets will still aggregate on the replacement. These could become emboli, therefore increasing risk of stroke.
   ii. He will require an antibacterial agent, preferably penicillin (unless he is allergic) for prophylaxis, because invasive procedures provide a portal of entry for bacteria that may then colonize the prosthetic valve, causing infective endocarditis.

70. (p. 341) group A β-hemolytic streptococci
71. (p. 341)
   those between the age of 5 and 15 years
   economically disadvantaged individuals
   those living in crowded conditions: institutions, major urban centers, large families in small cramped quarters
72. (pp. 341-342, Fig. 18-28) An acute systemic inflammatory condition resulting from abnormal immune reaction of an untreated infection, usually β-hemolytic streptococci. Results in acute cardiac inflammation involving one or more layers of the heart: pericarditis, myocarditis, and/or endocarditis. Other sites of inflammation include large joints, particularly in the legs; migratory polyarthritis; nonpruritic skin rash; nontender subcutaneous nodules on the extensor surfaces of wrists, elbows, knees, or ankles; and inflammation of the basal nuclei in the brain, causing involuntary jerky movements. Rheumatic heart disease can develop years later.
73. (pp. 341-342)
   i. general manifestations of inflammation: low-grade fever, leukocytosis, malaise, anorexia, and fatigue
   ii. pericarditis: inflammation of the outer layer of the heart; may include effusion
   iii. myocarditis: inflammation develops as localized lesions in the heart muscle, called Aschoff bodies
   iv. endocarditis: inflammation of the inner lining of the heart, especially the valves, which become edematous; verrucae (small wartlike lesions) form
   v. polyarthritis: migratory inflammation of many joints, especially in the legs
   vi. skin manifestations: erythema marginatum (red macules or papules)
   vii. subcutaneous nodules: nontender lesions on the extensor surfaces of wrists, elbows, and knees

viii. chorea: inflammation of the basal nuclei in the brain causing involuntary jerky movements of the face, arms, and legs

74. (p. 341) Endocarditis may lead to permanent scarring of heart valves, which leads to rheumatic heart disease. If rheumatic heart disease develops, the individual is now at high risk for infective endocarditis.

75. (p. 342) CBC and serology for identifying leukocytosis and anemia; monitoring antistreptolysin O antibody titer; ECG to identify characteristic changes

76. (p. 342)

Medication	Effects	Example
Antibiotics	Eradicate bacteria and prevent further infection	Penicillin (first choice unless patient is allergic)
NSAIDs	Decrease acute inflammation to prevent heart complications Relieve joint symptoms Lower fever	ASA Ibuprofen
Corticosteroids	Decrease immune response and acute inflammation to prevent heart complications	Prednisone
Antipyretics	Decrease fever	ASA Ibuprofen Acetaminophen
Antiarrhythmics	Improve efficiency of heart function and prevent complications	Metoprolol Nifedipipine Digoxin
Muscle relaxants	Decrease muscle spasms	Diazepam

77. (Think About) restriction of physical activities; maintenance of nutrition and hydration

78. (pp. 341-342, Figs. 18-28 and 18-29) Rheumatic fever is an acute, inflammatory disorder caused by abnormal immune response, following an infection by group A β-hemolytic streptococci. Rheumatic heart disease is a complication of rheumatic fever that involves permanent scarring of one or more heart valves; the individual is at high risk of infective endocarditis. Scar tissue in the myocardium may cause arrhythmias.

79. (p. 341) mitral valve, followed by aortic

80. (Think About, p. 342) Damaged heart valve stimulates platelet aggregation, leading to increased risk of emboli and stroke.

81. (p. 343) Damaged endocardial surface provides environment for bacterial colonization.

82. (p. 343) There are two predisposing factors for subacute infective endocarditis: damaged endocardium and portal of entry for bacteria or other organisms. Someone with RHD has damaged heart valves, and the invasive procedure provides the portal of entry.

83. (p. 340) Despite replacement of damaged valve, platelets will still aggregate on the replacement. These could become emboli, therefore increasing risk of stroke.

84. (p. 343) subacute: defective heart valves infected by organisms with low virulence; acute: normal valves attacked by highly virulent pathogens

85. (p. 343) Those with
a history of rheumatic heart disease
prosthetic heart valve(s)
recent stent insertion
renal dialysis
indwelling catheters
joint replacement within the past 2 years
immunosuppression or immunodeficiency
IV drug use

86. (p. 343)
infection of normal or defective heart valves
inflammation of the valves and formation of vegetations on the cusps
defective opening and closing of valves
potential for septic emboli causing infarction or infection
additional scarring and destruction of valve leaflets and chordae tendinea

87. (p. 343) Subacute infective endocarditis has an insidious onset. Various new heart murmurs are common. An initial low-grade fever and fatigue may be signs. Anorexia, splenomegaly, and Osler's nodes on the fingers are often present. There are signs of vascular occlusion or infection (abscesses)

185

in remote locations. An intermittent high fever (septicemia) may develop, and in severe cases, congestive heart failure develops. Acute endocarditis has a sudden onset with sudden spiked fever, chills, and drowsiness. Heart valves are badly damaged and may be torn, causing severe impairment of heart function. As in the subacute form, septic emboli may cause infarctions and abscesses in remote sites with corresponding signs and symptoms of infection.

88. (p. 344) blood culture—several samples are taken, preferably during a chill
89. (p. 344) Treatment includes antibacterials, preferably penicillin and drugs to support heart function; antiarrhythmics, and cardiac glycosides.
90. (pp. 341-344)

	Rheumatic Fever	Infective Endocarditis
Causative agent(s)	Group A β-hemolytic streptococci	Acute *Staphylococcus aureus* (most common) Subacute *Streptococcus viridans* (most common) Gram-negative bacilli Enterococci Fungi
Predisposing factors	Age: 5-15 Economically disadvantaged Living in crowded conditions	Damaged endocardium: rheumatic heart disease, previous endocarditis, congenital heart defects, prosthetic heart valves Portal of entry for microbes: IV drug users, indwelling catheters, recent joint replacement
Manifestations and complications	General: fever, leukocytosis, malaise, fatigue, anorexia Heart: pericarditis, myocarditis, endocarditis, tachycardia, heart murmur, arrhythmias, heart failure Polyarthritis Skin manifestations: rash Chorea Subcutaneous nodules Epistaxis Abdominal pain	General: fever, leukocytosis, fatigue, anorexia, elevated ESR Positive blood culture Change in heart murmur Septic emboli: Cough, dyspnea Arthralgia, arthritis Petechial hemorrhages in skin, mucosa, nail bed Chest pain Confusion, paralysis, stroke Blindness Hematuria Abdominal pain
Antibiotic of choice	Penicillin	Penicillin or other drug specific for causative agent
Prophylactic antibiotic coverage?	Not unless permanent heart valve problems (i.e., rheumatic heart disease); then amoxicillin	Yes—amoxicillin unless allergic

91. (pp. 312, 345) High blood pressure, when the systolic pressure is above 120 and the diastolic pressure is above 70 when an individual is at rest. Essential hypertension develops when blood pressure is consistently above 140/90 mm Hg. Men are more likely to have hypertension prior to age 55, after which women have a greater incidence. Differences in systolic and diastolic pressure increase with age, as the elasticity of arteries is lost.

92. (p. 345) Essential hypertension is idiopathic. Secondary hypertension results from renal or endocrine disease or pheochromocytoma.
93. (p. 345) nephrosclerosis, hyperaldosteronism, pheochromocytoma
94. (p. 345) hypertension that is uncontrollable, severe, and rapidly progressive with many complications and characterized by high diastolic pressure

95. (p. 346)
genetic factors—nonmodifiable
excessive alcohol intake—modifiable
high sodium intake—modifiable
obesity—modifiable
prolonged or recurrent stress—modifiable

96. (pp. 345-346, Fig. 18-31) There is an increase in arteriolar vasoconstriction, possibly due to increased susceptibility to various stimuli. There is a major increase in peripheral resistance, reducing the capacity of the system and increasing diastolic pressure. Decrease renal blood flow causes an increase in renin, angiotensin, and aldosterone secretion. Resulting increases in vasoconstriction and blood volume further increase blood pressure. Chronic hypertension causes arterial wall damage, sclerosis, and stenosis. Aneurysms or atheromas may form, reducing blood flow to involved area. There is ischemia and necrosis of involved tissues. The areas most frequently damaged are kidneys, brain, and retina. The end result of poorly con-trolled hypertension can be chronic renal failure, stroke, vision loss, or congestive heart failure.

97. (p. 346) It is often asymptomatic in the early stage, and initial symptoms are usually vague. Often the first indication is something dramatic like chest pain, heart attack, or stroke.

98. (pp. 345-346) Manifestations of early symptoms include headache on awakening, particularly in the occipital region; fatigue, dizziness, ringing in the ears; nosebleeds; shortness of breath on exertion (SOBOE); fainting; and failing vision. Manifestations of advanced symptoms include weakness, loss of vision, edema, congestive heart failure, angina pectoris, cerebrovascular accident, and renal failure.

99. (p. 346) Reduce salt intake, body weight, and stress and increase cardiovascular fitness.

100. (p. 347) patient compliance—i.e., willingness to consistently follow treatment plan

101. (Table 18-1, pp. 315-317, p. 346)

Type of Antihypertensive	Mechanism of Action and Effects	Adverse Effects	Examples
Diuretics	Increased excretion of sodium and water leading to decreased blood volume	Nausea, vomiting Orthostatic hypotension, dizziness Xerostomia Hypokalemia	Furosemide Hydrochlorothiazide
ACE inhibitors	Blocks formation of angiotensin II Decreased aldosterone secretion Prevent vasoconstriction	Headache Orthostatic hypotension, dizziness	Enalapril Ramipril Captopril Fosinopril
Calcium channel blockers	Vasodilatation Decrease myocardial conduction and contractility	Dizziness, fainting, headache Orthostatic hypotension Constipation Gingival hypertension	Nifedipine Amolodipine Diltiazem
β-Adrenergic blockers	Prevent increased heart rate in response to sympathetic nervous system and cholamines	Bradycardia Dizziness, fatigue Orthostatic hypotension Sexual dysfunction	Metoprolol Atenolol Propranolol Nadolol

102. (p. 347) orthostatic hypotension, dizziness; xerostomia

103. (p. 322, Table 18-1, p. 317)
platelet inhibitor: to prevent heart attacks and strokes
antihyperlidemic: to arrest or slow progression of atherosclerosis

104. (p. 348)
increasing fatigue and weakness in the legs
intermittent claudication
sensory impairment
weak peripheral pulse distal to the occlusion

marked pallor or cyanosis when legs elevated; redness when they are dangling
skin that is dry and hairless
toenails that are thick and hard
poorly perfused extremities that are cold

105. (p. 348)
reduction in serum cholesterol levels
platelet inhibitors or anticoagulants to reduce thrombosis
smoking cessation
exercise program
maintaining dependent position for the legs

peripheral vasodilators
surgical procedures to increase blood flow
preventive measures to avoid skin trauma
antibiotics for gangrenous ulcers

amputations when necessary to prevent infection spread; relieve pain
106. (pp. 348-349)

	Buerger's Disease	Raynaud's Disease
High-risk groups	Males before 35 years of age Smoking Genetics	Young women Certain preexisting conditions such as lupus
Etiology	Inflammatory disorder ? Abnormal immune response	Idiopathic
Vessels involved	Primarily medium-size and small arteries of legs and arms Sometimes adjacent vein involvement	Small arteries and arterioles in fingers and less frequently toes
Pathophysiology	Inflammation leading to thrombosis and fibrosis resulting in vascular occlusion and ulceration, ultimately to gangrene	Periodic vasospasm leads to temporary ischemia that, if severe, results in paraesthesia and ulcerations
Manifestations	Severe pain, even at rest Cyanosis Changes in nails and skin texture Ulceration	Pallor, numbness, and cyanosis, followed by redness and throbbing pain Long term, interference withmanual dexterity

107. (p. 349) localized dilatation of an arterial wall
108. (p. 349) Causes include atherosclerosis, trauma (particularly automobile accidents), syphilis, and congenital defects.
109. (p. 349) rupture, leading to moderate bleeding or severe hemorrhage and death; or thrombus may develop in the aneurysm, causing obstruction
110. (p. 350) inherent weakness or defect in vein walls or valves (familial tendency); long periods of standing
111. (p. 350)
superficial varicosities on the legs appear as irregular, purplish, bulging veins in the legs
edema in the feet
fatigue and aching in the legs are common
shiny, pigmented, and hairless skin
ulcers may develop
112. (p. 351) thrombophlebitis: development of a thrombus in a vein in which inflammation is present; phlebothrombosis: spontaneous thrombus development in the absence of inflammation
113. (pp. 351-352)
blood stasis or sluggish blood flow
endothelial injury
increased blood coagulability
114. (p. 352)
exercise
elevation of legs
compression or elastic stockings
115. (p. 327; see also Chapter 19) Pulmonary embolus is a blood clot (or sometimes other material) that

blocks a pulmonary artery or one of its branches. It typically originates in leg veins due to thrombophlebitis.
116. (p. 352) hypotension resulting from a decreased circulating blood volume, resulting in decreased tissue perfusion and general hypoxia
117. (pp. 352-353, Fig. 18-36, p. 355)
SNS and adrenal medulla stimulated to increase the heart rate, force of contractions, and systemic vasoconstriction
renin secreted to activate angiotensin, a vasoconstrictor, and aldosterone to increase blood volume (sodium and water retention)
increased ADH to promote water reabsorption in the kidneys and thereby increase blood volume
glucocorticoids secreted to help stabilize the vascular system
acidosis stimulates respirations, increasing oxygen supply
118. (pp. 355-357, Table 18-5)
thirst, anxiety, and restlessness, because SNS is quickly stimulated by hypotension
Compensation follows as vasoconstriction shunts blood from the viscera and skin to the vital areas.
Progressive signs include lethargy, weakness and faintness, and metabolic acidosis due to decrease in blood flow and blood pressure. Metabolic acidosis may result as anaerobic metabolism increases lactic acid secretion.
119. (pp. 355-357, Figs. 18-36 and 18-37) If shock is prolonged, the body's responsiveness diminishes as

oxygen supply decreases and wastes accumulate. Compensated metabolic acidosis progresses to decompensated acidosis (see also Chapter 6). There is depression of the central nervous system, loss of cell metabolism, and reduction in effectiveness of medications. The progression to irreversible shock results in acute renal failure due to tubular ischemia and necrosis and ARDS.

120. (p. 357, including Emergency Treatment box)
Place patient in supine position.
Cover and keep warm.
Call 911.
Administer oxygen if possible.
Determine underlying cause and treat if possible; e.g., pressure for bleeding.

121. (Table 18-4, p. 353, Fig. 18-35, p. 354)

Type of Shock	Etiology	Specific Manifestations	Specific Treatment
Hypovolemic or hemorrhagic	Blood or plasma loss Dehydration: vomiting, diarrhea "Third spacing"	Bleeding Burns Dysphagia, nausea, vomiting, diarrhea Ascites Signs of peritonitis	Blood or plasma transfusions Fluid and electrolyte replacement Treat specific cause, e.g., measures to stop bleeding
Cardiogenic	Myocardial infarction Arrhythmias	Warning signs of infarction ECG changes	Antiarrhythmic agents ECG monitoring See treatment of myocardial infarction
Anaphylactic	Severe allergic or hypersensitivity reaction lead to generalized vasodilation	Severe dyspnea, wheezing, chest tightness Pruritis, urticaria (hives), tingling Flushing, feeling of warmth	Epinephrine IM or IV (Epi-Pen) Corticosteroids Antihistamines
Septic	Severe, overwhelming infection	High fever, possibly with chills Warm, flushed, dry skin Rapid, strong pulse Hyperventilation	Antibacterial Corticosteroids Antipyretics
Neurogenic (syncope)	Pain or fear Emotional upset (unpleasant sight or smell)	Sudden vertigo and loss of consciousness Flushed, warm skin	Spirits of ammonia "smelling salts" Lower head Remove stimulus

122. (pp. 304+)
i. ascites: right-sided heart failure
ii. positive Homan's sign: thrombophlebitis
iii. ECG changes: myocardial infarction; arrhythmias
iv. positive blood cultures: rheumatic fever, endocarditis
v. claudication: thrombophlebitis, Buerger's disease
vi. hemoptysis: heart failure
vii. heart murmur: congenital defects, rheumatic fever, rheumatic heart disease, tetralogy of Fallot, septal defects, valvular defects—stenosis and regurgitation
viii. elevated cardiac enzymes: myocardial infarction
ix. subcutaneous nodules: rheumatic fever

x. pulmonary edema: left-sided heart failure, mitral stenosis, mitral regurgitation

123. (Table 18-1, pp. 315-317, 346)
i. calcium channel blockers: antihypertensive, antiarrhythmic, prophylactic antianginal
ii. nitroglycerin: antianginal—prophylactic or acute
iii. penicillin: scarlet fever, rheumatic fever, rheumatic heart disease
iv. β-adrenergic blockers: antihypertensive, antiarrhythmic, prophylactic antianginal
v. digoxin: heart failure, antiarrhythmic
vi. diuretics: heart failure, hypertension
vii. antiarrhythmics: arrhythmias, post–myocardial infarction, rheumatic fever
viii. ACE inhibitors: antihypertensive

CHAPTER 19

Respiratory Disorders

1. (Fig. 19-8, p. 377) otitis media, sinusitis, pneumonia
2. (pp. 377-379, Table 19-3, p. 378)

	Croup (Laryngotracheobronchitis)	Epiglottitis	Bronchiolitis
Usual age	3 months to 3 years	3-7 years	2-12 months
Cause	Virus	*Haemophilus influenzae*	Virus: RSV
Onset	Gradual	Rapid	Gradual
Pathology	Inflammation of mucosa of larynx and trachea obstructs airway	Supraglottic inflammation and swelling of epiglottis obstruct airway	Inflammation of mucosa of bronchioles obstructs small passages
Significant manifestations	Hoarse, barking cough Inspiratory stridor Restlessness	Drooling, dysphagia High fever, appears ill Rapid respirations and pulse Tripod position	Increasing dyspnea Paroxysmal cough, wheezing Chest retractions flared nostrils
Treatment	Cool, moisturized air from a humidifier, shower, or croup tent	Oxygen and antimicrobial therapy with intubation or tracheotomy if necessary	Supportive or symptomatic with monitoring of blood gases in severe cases

3. (Fig. 19-9, p. 380, Table 19-4, p. 381)

	Lobar Pneumonia	Bronchial Pneumonia	Interstitial Pneumonia
Causative agent	*Streptococcus pneumoniae*	Multiple bacteria	Influenza virus Mycoplasma
Onset	Sudden and acute	Insidious	Variable
Distribution within lungs	All of one or two lobes	Scattered small patches	Scattered small patches
Pathophysiology	Inflammation of alveolar wall and leakage of cells, fibrin, and fluid into alveoli causing consolidation	Inflammation and purulent exudate in alveoli often arising from prior pooled secretions or irritation	Interstitial inflammation around alveoli Necrosis of bronchial epithelium
Manifestations	High fever and chills Productive cough with rusty sputum Rales progressing to absence of breath sounds in affected lobes	Mild fever Productive cough with yellow-green sputum Dyspnea	Variable fever, headache Aching muscles Nonproductive hacking cough
Treatment	Antibacterial medication in combination with fluids, drugs to reduce fever and oxygen Pneumococcal vaccine is recommended for the elderly and those at risk of other disease	Antibacterial medications	Erythromycin or tetracycline

4. (p. 382) PCP is an atypical pneumonia that occurs as an opportunistic and often fatal infection in patients with AIDS. It may also cause pneumonia in premature infants. The etiologic agent is a fungus that is inhaled and attaches to alveolar cells, causing necrosis and diffuse interstitial inflammation. Onset is marked by dyspnea and a nonproductive cough.

5. (pp. 382-383) SARS-CoV (SARS-associated coronavirus) is the microbial agent responsible for SARS. It is transmitted by respiratory droplets during close contact.

6. (p. 383) Flulike symptoms are present for 3 to 7 days followed several days later by a dry cough and marked dyspnea. By day 7, chest radiographs indicate spreading patchy areas of interstitial congestion and severe hypoxia; there may be thrombocytopenia, lymphopenia, and elevated liver enzymes (due to viral damage). The final stage is severe, sometimes fatal respiratory distress.

7. (p. 383)
   stage 1: fever, headache, myalgia, diarrhea
   stage 2: nonproductive cough, severe dyspnea, hypoxia
   stage 3: severe hypoxia, respiratory and metabolic acidosis

8. (p. 383) medications: ribaviron (antiviral) and GC-methylprednisolone; oxygen with mechanical ventilation

9. (Think About, pp. 375-383) It is difficult to control the spread of an unidentified causative agent because the type of microbe has not been identified as bacterial, viral, or fungal. The routes of transmission may not be known. The agent's sensitivity to antimicrobial medications is not known. The usual course of the infection (i.e., complications and prognosis) may be unknown.

10. (p. 383) acid-fast, aerobic, slow-growing bacillus that is resistant to drying and many disinfectants

11. (p. 383) The cell wall prevents digestion and destruction by defensive cells.

12. (pp. 385-386) Those whose resistance is lowered because of immunodeficiency, malnutrition, alcoholism, conditions of war, or chronic disease. There may be a genetic susceptibility. Children are vulnerable, as are the homeless. Patients with AIDS are also at high risk.

13. (pp. 383-385, Figs. 19-11 and 19-12) In the primary infection, the pathogen is engulfed by macrophages and causes local inflammatory reaction, usually on the periphery of the upper lobe. Some bacilli migrate to the lymph nodes, activating a type IV hypersensitivity response. Lymphocytes and macrophages cluster to form a granuloma at the site of inflammation. The granuloma contains the bacilli, some of which remain alive, forming a tubercle. Caseation necrosis develops in the center of the tubercle. The secondary infection is the active infection. It often arises years after primary infection due to decreased host resistance. Tissue necrosis and cavitation occur,

forming a large open area in the lung and erosion into the bronchi and blood vessels. Hemoptysis is common. Infection may spread to other body systems, and bacilli may infect sputum.

14. (p. 384) Ghon tubercle is the core of caseation necrosis, surrounded by lymphocytes and macrophages. It is eventually walled off by fibrous tissue and usually becomes calcified.

15. (p. 385) Primary tuberculosis is asymptomatic. Secondary infection has an insidious onset with vague symptoms of anorexia, malaise, fatigue, and weight loss; afternoon low-grade fever and night sweats; prolonged and increasingly severe cough; and productive, purulent sputum, often containing blood.

16. (p. 384) rapidly progressive form in which multiple granulomas affect large areas of the lungs with rapid dissemination via the bloodstream; resistant to treatment

17. (p. 386) with chest radiograph and sputum specimen

18. (pp. 384 and 386; see also Chapter 3, Type IV Delayed Hypersensitivity) The Mantoux test is the tuberculin test. A positive skin test does NOT mean the person has active TB. It means that there has been adequate exposure to cause a hypersensitivity reaction.

19. (p. 386) isoniazid (INH); rifampin; ethambutol; pyrazinamide; streptomycin; multiple drugs required in order to prevent the development of resistant strains; 3 months to 1 year or possibly longer, depending upon the health of the individual—e.g., someone who also has full-blown AIDS will probably take TB medications for the rest of his life.

20. (p. 386) An individual will become noncontagious when sputum is negative for microbes, usually about 1 to 2 months. Drugs are prescribed for a longer period of time to ensure eradication of the infection.

21. (Think About)
   those whose skin test has converted from negative to positive within the past 2 years
   those who have radiographic changes consistent with tuberculosis, even if their sputum is negative
   anyone who is living with an individual with active tuberculosis
   individuals who have immunosuppression due to disease or medications
   people who are HIV positive or have full-blown AIDS
   persons with hematological cancer

22. (p. 386) Isoniazid is usually prescribed for 1 year.

23. (Think About 19-7, p. 386) have regular skin tests and, if the test is positive, regular chest radiographs; maintain host resistance (adequate rest, nutrition)

24. (Think About 19-7, p. 386)
   date of skin test
   Was he vaccinated against TB as a child?
   Has he had any known contact with person who has TB or a history of TB?

Did he have a follow-up chest radiograph or sputum specimen for AFB?

Did the doctor prescribe medication?

Is he taking the medication? How long has he been taking the medication?

25. (Think About 19-7, p. 386)

Was TB actually diagnosed, or was it a positive skin test?

Was he prescribed medications?

How long were the medications prescribed for?

Did he actually take the medication at the intervals and for the time period prescribed?

When was his last chest radiograph?

26. (p. 386; see also Chapter 7, Table 7-1) an autosomal recessive inherited disorder

27. (See Chapter 7, Fig. 7-4, p. 165) Both parents are heterozygous—i.e., carriers of cystic fibrosis. There is a 25% probability that the baby's siblings will have CF.

28. (See Chapter 7, Fig. 7-4, p. 165) There is a 50% probability that the child will have CF and a 50% probability that he will be a carrier.

29. (pp. 386-387, Fig. 19-13) Cystic fibrosis is a common genetic disorder involving a protein in chloride ion transport in cell membranes. This defect in the exocrine glands causes thick secretions, such as tenacious mucus. Primary effects are seen in lungs and pancreas where mucus blocks passages. In the lungs, there is progressive destruction of lung tissue and atelectasis, and infections are common. Bronchiectasis and emphysematous changes develop. Eventually, respiratory failure or cor pulmonale develops. In the digestive tract, the first indication of abnormality may be meconium ileus in newborns. Pancreatic blockage leads to digestive enzyme deficit in the intestines. Malabsorption and malnutrition develop. Potential pancreatic glandular tissue damage results in diabetes mellitus in some individuals. Biliary obstruction leads to fat and fat-soluble vitamin malabsorption and deficiencies. Ultimately, the general state of malabsorption, malnutrition, and dehydration develops. The salivary glands are mildly affected, causing patchy fibrosis. Sweat glands are affected, producing high chloride sweat and potential electrolyte disturbance in hot weather or during strenuous exercise. Obstructions in male (vas deferens) and female (cervix) reproductive systems lead to sterility or infertility.

30. (pp. 387-388) meconium ileus at birth; salty skin; signs of malabsorption: steatorrhea, abdominal distention, and failure to gain weight; chronic cough and frequent respiratory infections; progressive hypoxia, fatigue and exercise intolerance; growth failure

31. (p. 388) electrolyte analysis of sweat; stool analysis for fat content and trypsin; pulmonary function tests, radiographs and blood gases; genetic analysis

32. (pp. 388-389): interdisciplinary team approach; replacement therapy for pancreatic enzymes and bile salts; specialized diet; measures to avoid dehydration; chest physiotherapy; bronchodilators and humidifiers; aggressive treatment of infections; oxygen therapy for advanced disease

33. (p. 389) Individuals with CF on average live into early adulthood. Death is usually brought on through infections and respiratory or heart failure.

34. (p. 389) Venous return and lymphatics bring tumor cells from many distant sites to the heart and then into the pulmonary circulation.

35. (p. 390) cigarette smoking, especially heavy smokers; second-hand smoke; COPD; genetic factors; occupational or industrial exposure to carcinogens

36. (p. 390) obstruction of airflow by tumor growth into the bronchus; inflammation surrounding the tumor stimulates cough and predisposes secondary infection; pleural effusion, hemothorax, pneumothorax due to inflammation or erosion of pleura; paraneoplastic syndrome; general systemic effects of cancer

37. (pp. 390-391) Early signs related to respiratory involvement include persistent productive cough, dyspnea, and wheezing; radiographic changes signifying pneumonia; hemoptysis; pleural involvement—effusion; pneumothorax or hemothorax; chest pain; hoarseness; facial or arm edema and headache due to compression of superior vena cava; dysphagia; and atelectasis. Systemic signs include weight loss, anemia, and fatigue. Paraneoplastic syndrome is indicated by signs of specific endocrine disorder. Signs of metastasis depend on site, e.g., bone.

38. (p. 391)

surgical resection or lobectomy

chemotherapy

radiation

photodynamic therapy

39. (p. 391) passage of food or fluid, vomitus, drugs, or other foreign material into the trachea and lungs

40. (p. 392) young children; children with congenital anomalies such as cleft palate; any individual with depressed swallowing or gag reflex; e.g., following anesthesia or stroke or comatose patients; individuals who eat or drink while lying down or talking while eating

41. (pp. 391-392)

solid objects lodge in the airway and totally block airflow at that point

large objects may occlude the trachea and block all airflow

solid objects lodging in a bronchus lead to nonaeration and collapse of the area distal to the obstruction (see Fig. 19-23, p. 407)

ball-valve effect of solid object: air flows in on inspiration, airway closes on expiration

swelling of some foods (beans) that become more firmly lodged

sharp pointed objects, like bone fragments, may traumatize mucosa and cause inflammation that further adds to the airway barrier

fatty or irritating solids such as peanuts cause inflammation, creating edema and further impeding airflow

irritating liquids (e.g., vomitus, alcohol) cause severe inflammation, narrowing airways, and increased secretions; if alveoli involved, can impair gaseous exchange: called chemical or *aspiration* pneumonia
complications include respiratory distress syndrome, pulmonary abscess, systemic affects of aspirated solvents

42. (p. 392) coughing and choking with marked dyspnea; stridor and hoarseness (upper airway obstruction); wheezing (liquids); tachycardia and tachypnea; nasal flaring, chest retractions; inability to speak or make a sound (total obstruction of larynx or trachea)

43. (Emergency Treatment Box, p. 393) Stand behind the victim with encircling arms, position a fist, thumb side against the abdomen, just below the sternum, place the other hand over the fist, and thrust forcefully inward and upward.

44. (p. 393) a disease that involves periodic episodes of severe but reversible bronchial obstruction

45. (p. 393) Extrinsic asthma involves acute episodes triggered by a type I hypersensitivity reaction to an inhaled antigen. A familial history of other allergies is common. Onset usually occurs in children. Intrinsic asthma usually occurs in adulthood. Other types of stimuli target hyperresponsive tissues in the airway, initiating the acute attack. These stimuli include respiratory infections, exposure to cold, exercise, certain drugs such as aspirin, stress, and inhalation of irritants such as cigarette smoke.

46. (p. 393)
respiratory infections
exposure to cold
exercise
certain drugs, such as aspirin
stress
inhalation of irritants such as cigarette smoke

47. (p. 393, Fig. 19-17, p. 394) an acute allergic response to stimuli affecting the bronchioles, resulting in inflammation of the mucosa with edema, contraction of smooth muscle (bronchoconstriction), and increased thick mucus secretion in the air passages,

with resulting airway obstruction and interference with airflow and oxygen supply

48. (p. 394)
hyperinflation of the lung, with increased residual volume
atelectasis
respiratory and metabolic acidosis
status asthmaticus
chronic asthma and obstructive lung disease

49. (p. 396)
cough, dyspnea, tightness in the chest, and agitation as airway obstruction increases; cannot talk
wheezing
rapid and labored breathing
coughing up thick and tenacious mucus
tachycardia and perhaps pulsus paradoxus
hypoxia
respiratory alkalosis, initially due to hyperventilation
respiratory acidosis, in time, due to air trapping
marked fatigue causes reduced respiratory effort and weaker cough
metabolic acidosis
severe respiratory distress; hypoventilation leading to hypoxemia and respiratory acidosis
respiratory failure: decreasing responsiveness, cyanosis

50. (p. 396)
avoidance of triggering stimuli
a program of desensitization or "allergy shots" for allergens that cannot be avoided (e.g., house dust)
good ventilation: at home, school, work
conditioning exercises to strengthen muscles of respiration and improve cardiovascular fitness (swimming is particularly good as long as the water is not too cold)
relaxation techniques to help cope with stressful situations and hopefully to avoid precipitating an attack
flu vaccinations or inoculations
avoidance of individuals with respiratory infections

51. (p. 396)

Drug Group	Action and Effects	Adverse Effects	Example and Route
Bronchodilators	Relax bronchial smooth muscle leading to bronchodilation	Tachycardia, palpitations CNS stimulation: tremors, insomnia Stinging sensation in mouth	Inhalants Albuterol or salbutamol (Ventolin) Metaproterenol (Alupent)
Corticosteroids	Decrease inflammation Decrease the immune response (hypersensitivity)	Oral fungal (candidial) infections with inhalants Cushing's with oral administration	Inhalation: beclomethasone (Beclovent) Oral: prednisone
Histamine release inhibitors	Inhibit release of histamine from sensitized mast cells Decrease the number of eosinophils	Rare	Inhalation Cromlyn (Intal)
Leukotriene receptor antagonists	Block inflammatory response in order to prevent bronchoconstriction and mucus production	Rarely, GI distress	Inhalation Montelukast (Singulair) Zafirlukast (Accolade)

52. (p. 396) Bronchodilators can be used during an acute asthmatic attack because their mechanism of action is to prevent or decrease an allergic response or inflammation. If an individual is experiencing an attack, the chemical mediators have already been released and the inflammation is already happening.

53. (p. 396) histamine release inhibitors

54. (Think About, p. 396) epinephrine and oxygen

55. (Think About, pp. 393-397)
How frequent are his asthmatic attacks?
When was the last one?
What are the triggering stimuli for an acute episode?
How long do they usually last?
What is the treatment he uses during bronchospasm?
Has he had any emergencies when he had to seek medical help?

56. (p. 397, Table 19-5) Smoking is the leading causative factor. Contributing factors include cystic fibrosis and bronchiectasis; many occupational lung diseases such as silicosis, asbestosis, farmer's lung, and industrial/urban pollution.

57. (pp. 400-401) Both conditions are characterized by hypoxia—this stimulates release of erythropoietin by the kidneys, which in turn stimulates increased production of red blood cells

58. (p. 398) destruction of pulmonary alveolar walls and septa, leading to large permanently inflated alveolar air spaces

59. (p. 398)
loss of surface area for gas exchange
loss of pulmonary capillaries, affecting perfusion and diffusion of gases
loss of elasticity, affecting ability of lung to recoil on expiration
altered ventilation-perfusion ratio

decreased support for other pulmonary structures such as the small bronchi, leading to further collapse and obstruction of airflow during expiration

60. (pp. 400-401) Hyperventilation is a compensatory mechanism that alone helps maintain adequate oxygen levels until late in the disease; therefore, the patient's color is normal (i.e., pink), unlike in many respiratory disorders that are characterized by hypoxia and cyanosis.

61. (pp. 398, 400)
barrel chest
pneumothorax
frequent infections
pulmonary hypertension and cor pulmonale
clubbed fingers
secondary polycythemia

62. (p. 398) Hypercapnia develops, resulting in respiratory acidosis. Hypoxia leads to metabolic acidosis. Blood pH decreases.

63. (p. 398) Hypoxia becomes the driving force for respiration as respiratory control adapts to chronic hypercapnia.

64. (p. 398) Barrel chest refers to the hyperinflation of lungs that leads to increased anterior-posterior diameter of chest. The chest appears like a barrel. The condition develops because accessory muscles of expiration hypertrophy.

65. (p. 400)
avoidance of respiratory irritants and sources of infections
smoking cessation
immunization against influenza and pneumonia
pulmonary rehabilitation
nutrition counseling: maintenance of adequate nutrition and hydration

bronchodilators, antimicrobials, and oxygen therapy when needed

lung reduction surgery

66. (p. 401) Following chronic irritation of the bronchi, the mucosa is inflamed and swollen; there is hypertrophy and hyperplasia of the mucous glands and increased secretions and fibrosis and thickening of the bronchial wall and further obstruction. Secretions pool distal to the obstruction and are difficult to remove; oxygen levels are low; and cyanosis may occur during coughing episodes.

67. (p. 401) constant productive cough

68. (p. 401) Hypoxia is characteristic feature, particularly during coughing episodes. This results in poor color or cyanosis. Pulmonary congestion and cor pulmonale also commonly occur with chronic bronchitis, resulting in peripheral edema. Thus there is a designation as a "blue bloater" as opposed to someone with emphysema, a "pink puffer."

69. (p. 401) Therapeutic interventions include reducing exposure to irritants, prompt treatment of infections, influenza and pneumonia vaccination, and use of expectorants, bronchodilators, chest therapy, low-flow oxygen, and nutritional supplementation.

70. (Table 19-5, p. 397)

	Asthma	Emphysema	Chronic Bronchitis
Etiology and predisposing factor	Family history of allergies Sedentary lifestyle Air pollution Obesity	Smoking Air pollution Genetic factor	Smoking Air pollution
Location	Small bronchi, bronchioles	Alveoli	Bronchi
Pathophysiology	Inflammation, bronchoconstriction, increased mucus produced; obstruction; repeat attacks lead to damage	Destruction of alveolar walls; loss of elasticity impaired expiration, barrel chest, hyperinflation	Increased mucous glands and secretions; inflammation and infection; obstruction
Manifestations	Cough, dyspnea, wheezing, thick, tenacious mucus	Some coughing, marked dyspnea	Early constant cough, some dyspnea, large amounts of purulent sputum
Complications	Some infections; cyanosis if status asthmaticus	Some infections Cor pulmonale: sometimes, late	Cyanosis; frequent infections Cor pulmonale
Therapeutic Interventions	Avoidance of triggering stimuli A program of desensitization or "allergy shots" for allergens that cannot be avoided (e.g., house dust) Good ventilation: at home, school, work Conditioning exercises to strengthen muscles of respiration and improve cardiovascular fitness Fitness (swimming is particularly good as long as the water is not too cold) Relaxation techniques to help cope with stressful situations and hopefully to avoid precipitating an attack Flu vaccinations or inoculations Avoidance of individuals with respiratory infections	Avoidance of respiratory irritants and sources of infections Smoking cessation Immunization against influenza and pneumonia Pulmonary rehabilitation Nutrition counseling: maintenance of adequate nutrition and hydration Bronchodilators, antimicrobials, and oxygen therapy when needed Lung reduction surgery	Reducing exposure to irritants Prompt treatment of infections Influenza and pneumonia vaccination Use of expectorants, bronchodilators Chest therapy Low-flow oxygen and nutritional supplementation

71. (p. 403) Causes include inflammation in the lungs, increasing capillary permeability; plasma protein levels are low, decreasing plasma osmotic pressure; pulmonary hypertension, increasing hydrostatic pressure.

72. (pp. 403-404, Fig. 19-21) Pulmonary edema occurs when excess fluid develops in the alveolar tissue. This fluid interferes with gaseous exchange, leading to severe hypoxemia. This accumulation of fluid interferes with the action of surfactant, leading to difficulty in expansion of lungs, which ultimately collapse.

73. (p. 403) Manifestations include cough, orthopnea, and rales; hemoptysis as congestion increases; frothy sputum; dyspnea; cyanosis due to increasing hypoxemia.

74. (p. 403) Sputum becomes frothy when air mixes with secretions and becomes blood-tinged due to ruptured capillaries in the lungs.

75. (p. 403) When placed in a supine position, the fluid that has accumulated in the bases of the lungs starts to shift into the upper lobes. Venous return to the heart and lungs is increased when in a supine position. The individual feels a sense of suffocation. This is called orthopnea.

76. (p. 404) Causative factors must be treated and supportive care such as oxygen therapy is provided; positive pressure mechanical ventilation may be necessary in severe cases. Upper body is elevated. Diuretics may be given to reduce fluid.

77. (p. 404) a blood clot or mass of material that obstructs the pulmonary artery or a branch of it

78. (pp. 404, 406) Most pulmonary emboli originate in the deep veins, primarily in the legs. Other potential sources include fat emboli from the bone marrow (fractures), vegetations resulting from endocarditis, amniotic fluid emboli, and tumor cell emboli.

79. (p. 406)
bedridden patients who have been immobile for long periods: e.g., hospitalized patients
anyone with leg trauma
mothers during childbirth
CHF patients
patients with dehydration or increased coagulability of the blood
cancer patients
airplane or automobile passengers who remain seated for prolonged periods of time

80. (pp. 405-406, Fig. 19-22) The effects depend on the size and location of the embolism. Small pulmonary emboli are frequently "silent" or asymptomatic. Multiple small emboli, however, equal the effect of a large embolus. Moderate-sized emboli usually cause respiratory impairment. Large emboli affect the cardiovascular system, causing right-sided heart failure and shock. Sudden death often occurs.

81. (p. 406) With a small embolus, manifestations include transient chest pain, cough, or dyspnea. With a larger embolus, manifestations include chest pain that increases with coughing or deep breathing, and tachypnea and dyspnea develop suddenly; later, hemoptysis and fever, anxiety and restlessness, pallor, and tachycardia occur. A massive emboli is characterized by severe crushing chest pain, low blood pressure, rapid, weak pulse, and loss of consciousness. Fat emboli are distinguished by development of acute respiratory distress, petechial rash on the trunk, and neurologic signs such as confusion and disorientation.

82. (p. 406) heparin or fibrinolytic agent

83. (pp. 401-402, 406-407, Fig. 19-23)

	Atelectasis	Bronchiectasis
Definition	Nonaeration or collapse of a lung or part of a lung	Irreversible dilation or widening of bronchi
Etiology	Total obstruction of an airway Compression of airway Increased alveolar surface tension Fibrotic tissue in lungs or pleura Following anesthesia	Complication of: Cystic fibrosis COPD Childhood infections Aspiration of foreign bodies
Complications	Permanent lung damage	Recurrent lung infections
Manifestations	Dyspnea; increased respirations Tachycardia Chest pain Abnormal chest expansion	Chronic productive cough Purulent sputum Rales and rhonchi Dyspnea, hemoptysis Foul breath Weight loss, anemia, fatigue

84. (pp. 408-410, Table 19-7, p. 409, Fig. 19-24, p. 411)

	Pleural Effusion	Pneumothorax
Definition	Excessive fluid in pleural cavity	Air in pleural cavity
Etiology	Inflammation	Spontaneous Rupture of a bleb (emphysema) Erosion by tumor Cavitation due to TB Puncture wound
Manifestations	Dyspnea Chest pain Increased heart and respiratory rates Absence of breath sounds in affected area	Increased, labored respirations with dyspnea Pain Asymmetrical chest movements Tachycardia

85. (pp. 410 and 412, Fig. 19-25) Flail chest results from fractures of the thorax (usually from falls and automobile accidents)—usually includes fractures of three to six ribs in two places or fracture of the sternum and a number of consecutive ribs resulting in *paradoxical movement* during inspiration and *mediastinal flutter* if injury is extensive.

86. (p. 416) Causes of acute respiratory failure include chronic conditions such as emphysema, combination of a chronic with an acute disorder such as emphysema complicated by pneumonia or pneumothorax, acute respiratory disorders such as chest trauma, pulmonary embolus, or acute asthma, and many neuromuscular diseases such as myasthenia gravis, amyotrophic lateral sclerosis, or muscular dystrophy.

87. (pp. 413-415)

	Infant Respiratory Distress Syndrome	Adult Respiratory Distress Syndrome
Etiology	Premature birth resulting in decreased surfactant	Systemic sepsis Prolonged shock Burns and smoke inhalation Aspiration
Pathophysiology	Lungs collapse with each expiration resulting in diffuse atelectasis, poor lung perfusion, and increased alveolar capillary permeability causing fluid and fibrin to leak into alveoli that decreases lung expansion and gas exchange	Damage to surfactant—producing cells and increased capillary permeability leading to diffuse atelectasis and decreased tidal volume and vital capacity and fluid accumulation in lungs, all of which predisposes to pneumonia
Manifestations	Respirations greater than 60/minute Nasal flaring; chest retractions Frothy sputum Decreased BP, cyanosis, depressed responsiveness Apnea	Marked dyspnea Tachycardia Decreased PO_2 Rales Frothy sputum Cyanosis Lethargy
Treatment	Corticosteroids to mother during labor Synthetic surfactant Mechanical ventilation and O_2	Treat underlying cause O_2 and mechanical ventilation

88. (pp. 402-410)
   a) air in the pleural cavity; iii. pneumothorax
   b) abnormal widening of the bronchii; iv. bronchiectasis
   c) excessive fluid in the pleural cavity; i. pleural effusion
   d) chronic disorders resulting from continued exposure to irritating particles; vi. pneumoconioses
   e) fungal infection of the lungs; v. histoplasmosis
   f) collapse of a portion of the lung; ii. atelectasis
89. (pp. 364-419)
   i. characterized by episodic bronchospasm: asthma
   ii. causes orthopnea: pulmonary edema
   iii. sputum often frothy and pink or blood-flecked: pulmonary edema
   iv. loss of alveolar walls and lung elasticity: emphysema
   v. caused by an acid-fast bacillus: tuberculosis
   vi. acute manifestations usually relieved by adrenergic agonists: asthma
   vii. occurs most commonly in immunosuppressed individuals: *Pneumocystis carinii* pneumonia
   viii. deficit of pancreatic digestive enzymes: cystic fibrosis
   ix. collapse of a lung or portion of a lung: atelectasis
   x. characterized by a constant productive cough: chronic bronchitis
   xi. potential complication of thrombophlebitis in leg veins: pulmonary embolus
   xii. inadequate production of surfactant: adult respiratory distress syndrome
   xiii. could result from a rib fracture: pneumothorax
   xiv. defect in chloride ion transport in cell membranes: cystic fibrosis
   xv. causes malabsorption of nutrients: cystic fibrosis
   xvi. may cause cavitation within lungs: tuberculosis
   xvii. abnormal dilation of the bronchi: bronchiectasis
   xviii. accumulation of fluid in the pleural cavity: pleurisy
   xix. characterized by caseation necrosis: tuberculosis
   xx. treated with leukotriene receptor antagonists: asthma

CHAPTER 20

Digestive System Disorders

1. a) drug used to decrease nausea and vomiting; iv. antiemetic
   b) formation of gallstones; x. cholelithiasis
   c) greasy, loose stools; i. steatorrhea
   d) loss of appetite; v. anorexia
   e) opportunistic oral fungal infection; viii. candidiasis
   f) outpouching of the mucosa in colon; xi. diverticulum
   g) tarry stools caused by bleeding; ii. melena
   h) difficulty swallowing; iii. dysphagia
   i) inflammation of the tissue surrounding the teeth; ix. gingivitis
   j) retention of feces; vii. impaction
   k) vomit containing blood; vi. hematemesis
2. (pp. 431-432)
   distention or irritation in digestive tract
   example: distention due to gas following abdominal surgery; constipation
   unpleasant sights or smells: sight of blood; odor of emesis or feces
   pain or stress: performance anxiety; postoperatively; going to dentist
   stimulation of vestibular apparatus in inner ear: motion sickness; amusement rides
   increased intracranial pressure: brain tumors, hydrocephalus; cerebral hemorrhage
   stimulation of chemoreceptor trigger zone: drugs, alcohol
3. (Table 20-3, p. 437)
   treat cause: e.g., analgesics for pain; laxatives or enema to relieve constipation
   antiemetic drugs
   sedatives
   antacids
   good ventilation to remove noxious odors
4. (p. 434)
   inadequate dietary fiber
   inadequate fluid intake
   failure to respond to the defecation reflex
   muscle weakness and inactivity
   neurologic disorders such as multiple sclerosis and spinal cord trauma
   drugs, such as opiates, CNS depressants, or anticholinergic drugs
   some antacids, iron medications, and bulk laxatives (with insufficient fluid intake)
   obstruction caused by tumors or strictures
5. (p. 436) increased fiber and fluid intake
6. (p. 444, Fig. 20-9, p. 445) Causes include
   esophageal fibrosis
   esophageal compression
   esophageal diverticulum
   congenital atresia of the esophagus
   congenital tracheoesophageal fistula
   neurologic damage to cranial nerves V, VII, IX, X, and XII
   achalasia
7. (p. 444, Fig. 20-10, p. 446) Part of the stomach is elevated and protrudes through an opening (hiatus) in the diaphragm into the thoracic cavity.
8. (p. 446) Manifestations include postprandial heartburn or pyrosis, a brief substernal burning sensation, often accompanied by sour taste; belching from regurgitation of gastric contents, especially when in a reclining position; and dysphagia.

9. (p. 446) Eliminating factors that reduce lower esophageal sphincter (LES) pressure, such as caffeine, fatty foods, alcohol, cigarette smoking, and certain drugs.

10. (p. 446) GERD is gastroesophageal reflux disease, the periodic flow of gastric contents into the esophagus. GERD is caused by hiatal hernia as well as other conditions that lower LES pressure or increase intra-abdominal pressure.

11. (pp. 436-437, Table 20-3, p. 437) antacids; histamine$_2$ (H$_2$ receptor) antagonist agents; proton pump inhibitors

12. (pp. 446-447) Acute gastritis is an inflammation of the gastric mucosa due to a variety of causes, including infection, food or drug allergy, ingestion of spicy or irritating food, excessive alcohol intake, ingestion of aspirin or other ulcerogenic drugs, ingestion of toxic substances, radiation, or chemotherapy. Acute gastroenteritis is inflammation of both the stomach and intestine usually caused by infection but may result from food or drug allergies.

13. (pp. 446-449)

	Acute Gastritis	Chronic Gastritis
Etiology	Infections Food allergies Spicy or irritating foods Drugs: aspirin; chemotherapy Ingestion of corrosive or toxic substances Radiation	Peptic ulcers Alcohol abuse Aging Pernicious anemia
Manifestations	Anorexia, nausea, vomiting Epigastric pain; cramps Hematemesis	Epigastric discomfort Intolerance of spicy foods

14. (Table 20-4, p. 448)

15. (p. 449, Figs. 20-11 and 20-12, pp. 450-451) Ulcers occur in proximal duodenum (most common), antrum of the stomach, and lower esophagus.

16. (p. 449) Factors include decreased mucosal resistance (gastric ulcers), excessive HCl or pepsin secretion (duodenal ulcers), and presence of bacterium *H. pylori*.

17. (pp. 449-451) Acid or pepsin penetrates the mucosal barrier. Tissues are exposed to continued damage because of acid diffusion into the gastric wall. Ulcers may erode more deeply into muscle layers and eventually perforate the wall. Inflammation surrounds the crater. Bleeding occurs when erosion invades a blood vessel. Bleeding may involve persistent loss of small amounts of blood or massive hemorrhage, depending on the size of the blood vessel involved.

18. (p. 451) Complications include
hemorrhage

perforation, resulting in chemical peritonitis and ultimately bacterial peritonitis
obstruction of the digestive tract due to scarring and stricture formation

19. (pp. 451-452) Manifestations include
epigastric burning or aching pain, usually 2 to 3 hours after meals and at night
heartburn, nausea, vomiting, and weight loss, especially after alcohol or irritating food
iron deficiency anemia or occult blood in the stool

20. (p. 452) Interventions include
drug therapy: usually combination of antimicrobials and acid reducers; coating agents or antacids for symptomatic relief
reducing exacerbating factors
vagotomy
partial gastrectomy or pyloroplasty in patients with perforated or bleeding ulcers

21. (pp. 444+; 452+; 467+; 469+; 477+)

	Etiology	Pathophysiology	Manifestations and Complications	Treatment
Esophagus	Chronic esophagitis Hiatal hernia Alcohol abuse Smoking	Circumferential or mass causing obstruction	Dysphagia	Surgery and radiation
Stomach	Diet: nitrates and smoked foods Genetics Chronic atrophic gastritis Polyps	Ulcerative-type lesion in mucosa or protruding mass or polyp Infiltrates into muscularis and serosa Spreads to liver and ovaries	Asymptomatic until late Indigestion Feelings of fullness Weight loss and fatigue Occult blood in stool Iron deficiency anemia	Combination therapy: surgery (gastric resection), chemotherapy, and radiation
Liver	Cirrhosis Hepatitis B and C Prolonged exposure to carcinogenic chemicals Metastases from abdominal organs	A mass that obstructs bile ducts and hepatic sinusoids Frequent site of metastases from other sites	Anorexia, vomiting, weight loss Jaundice Portal hypertension Splenomegaly	Chemotherapy
Pancreas	Cigarette smoking	Mass that obstructs ducts $\rightarrow$ congestion and inflammation $\rightarrow$ pancreatitis Early metastases	Abdominal pain Weight loss Jaundice	Surgery, radiation, and chemotherapy
Colorectal	Age: over 55 Familial multiple polyposis Ulcerative colitis Diet high in fat and red meat and low in fiber	May be polypoid May be ulcerative If circumferential may cause obstruction Metastasize to liver	Cramping Feeling of incomplete emptying Change bowel pattern and fecal consistency Occult blood in stool or melena	Surgery, both curative and palliative; may be accompanied by radiation and chemotherapy

22. (p. 456) women with high cholesterol levels in the bile; obesity, high cholesterol intake, and multi-parity; use of oral contraceptives or estrogen supplements; individuals with hemolytic anemia, alcoholic cirrhosis, or biliary tract infections

23. (p. 456) Manifestations include sudden severe waves of pain in the upper right quadrant of the abdomen or epigastric area, often radiating to the back or right shoulder; nausea and vomiting; increasing and then decreasing pain (if the stone moves on); and increasing pain followed by jaundice

24. (p. 456, Fig. 20-18, p. 458)
prehepatic; results from excessive destruction of RBCs, e.g., physiologic jaundice of some newborns, hemolytic anemias, transfusion reactions

intrahepatic: due to liver disease resulting in impaired uptake of bilirubin from the blood and decreased bilirubin conjugation; e.g., individuals with liver disease such as hepatitis or cirrhosis

posthepatic: obstruction of biliary flow due to congenital atresia of the bile ducts, cholelithiasis; inflammation or tumors of the liver

25. (p. 457) infectious mononucleosis or amebiasis; chemical or drug toxicity

26. (pp. 457-459, Table 20-5)

	Hepatitis A	Hepatitis B	Hepatitis C
Causative agent	HAV: RNA virus	HBV: double-stranded DNA virus	HCV: RNA virus
Transmission	Oral-fecal: "enteric"	Blood and body fluids	Blood and body fluids
High-risk groups	Individuals living in large institutions: prisons, nursing homes Children with poor toileting behavior Lower socioeconomic groups Travelers to developing countries Promiscuous oral-anal sex	IV drug users Those engaging in promiscuous, unprotected sex Those requiring hemodialysis Infants born to HBV+ mothers Those with multiple tattoos and body piercings Health care workers Recipients of blood and blood products before 1984	Same as for HBV, especially IV drug users Recipients of blood and blood products before 1990 Recipients of organ transplants Recipients of artificial insemination
Incubation period	2-6 weeks	1-6 months (average 60-90 days)	2 weeks to 6 months (average 6-9 weeks)
Severity of symptoms	Usually mild Most will be symptomatic, including jaundice	Occasionally severe, especially if coinfected with HDV	Often asymptomatic until many years after initial infection Only 25-30% develop jaundice
Duration of manifestations	2 months	4-12 weeks	2-12 weeks
Carrier state	None	Yes	Yes
Complications	Rare	Chronicity Hepatocellular carcinoma Cirrhosis and liver failure Fulminant hepatitis	Chronicity: more than 50% Hepatocellular cancer Cirrhosis and liver failure
Serological markers	Anti-HAV IgM: indicative of acute infection Anti-HAV IgG: indicative of past exposure	HBsAg: indicator of infection Anti-HBs: recovery and noninfectivity; effective protection HBeAg: marker of active infection Anti-HBe: signals onset of resolution Anti-HBc: marker of recent infection: NOT protective HBV DNA: indicator of infection	Anti-HCV: indicator of infection; NOT protective HCV RNA: indicator of infection
Medications	None	Chronic cases with abnormal liver function tests: Interferon alpha-2b Lamivudine	With elevated ALT: Interferon alpha-2b Ribaviron
Immunoglobul in vaccine	Yes	Yes	No

27. (p. 459) from virus-contaminated stool or food or fomites to hands to mouth and fomites (inanimate objects) by poor hygiene and unsanitary toilet practices (e.g., not washing hands after bowel movement); examples include

virus that has been excreted in stool of infected individual is ingested by another person

children with poor toileting behavior, particularly in large daycare centres

poor handwashing in nursing homes

eating shellfish from contaminated water

28. (p. 461) It is an incomplete RNA virus that requires the presence of HBV in order to replicate.

29. (Table 20-5, p. 459) by serological markers

30. (p. 461, Table 20-5, p. 459) fecal-oral route

31. (pp. 461-462) General manifestations include

preicteric stage: fatigue and malaise, anorexia and nausea, and general muscle aching; elevated serum levels of liver enzymes (AST, ALT)

icteric stage: jaundice; light-colored stool; dark urine and pruritic skin; tender, enlarged liver, causing mild aching pain; blood clotting times elevated in severe cases

posticteric stage: reduction in signs, may last for several weeks; depending on specific viral etiology

32. (Think About)

date of diagnosis

What type of hepatitis?

Has he ever been told not to give blood (may help to determine whether he had HBV or HCV if he is not sure)?

Is he a carrier?

Is he taking medications?

33. (p. 462) progressive destruction of liver tissue leading eventually to liver failure

34. (p. 463) Causes include

alcoholic liver disease

biliary cirrhosis: associated with immune disorders and those causing biliary obstruction such as stones or cystic fibrosis

postnecrotic cirrhosis: linked with chronic hepatitis or long-term exposure to toxic chemicals

metabolic: usually caused by storage disorders such as hemochromacytosis

35. (p. 463, Fig. 20-21) Liver demonstrates extensive diffuse fibrosis and loss of lobular organization. Nodules of regenerated hepatocytes may be present but are nonfunctional because the vascular network and biliary ducts are distorted. Fibrosis interferes with the blood supply. Bile may back up, causing ongoing inflammation and damage. Initial hepatomegaly is replaced by small, shrunken and scarred liver.

36. (pp. 463-464) Lost or impaired liver functions include

decreased removal and conjugation of bilirubin

decreased bile production

impaired digestion and absorption of nutrients, especially fats and fat-soluble vitamins

decreased production of blood-clotting factors and plasma proteins

impaired glucose/glycogen metabolism

inadequate storage of iron and vitamin B$_{12}$

decreased inactivation of hormones, such as aldosterone and estrogen

decreased removal of toxic substances from the blood

37. (Table 20-6, p. 464) Manifestations include fatigue, anorexia; ascites; general edema; esophageal varices, hemorrhoids; splenomegaly; anemia; leukopenia, thrombocytopenia; increased bleeding, purpura; hepatic encephalopathy, tremors, confusion, coma; gynecomastia, impotence, irregular menses; jaundice; and pruritis.

38. (p. 464, Fig. 20-22, p. 465) blockage of blood flow through the liver leading to high pressure in the portal veins

39. (p. 465, Figs. 20-22, 20-24, pp. 465-466)

ascites, splenomegaly, esophageal varices

impaired respiration

increased risk of peritonitis

impaired digestion and absorption

40. (p. 466-467) Interventions include supportive or symptomatic treatment, such as avoiding fatigue and exposure to infection; dietary restrictions on protein and sodium; high carbohydrate intake and vitamin supplementation; use of diuretics to balance serum electrolytes; paracentesis to remove excess fluid; albumin transfusions; antimicrobials such as neomycin to remove intestinal flora; surgery for esophageal varices; and liver transplantation.

41. (p. 469) gallstones and alcohol abuse

42. (pp. 468-469, Fig. 20-28) Pancreatitis results in premature activation of pancreatic enzymes inside the pancreatic duct followed by autodigestion of pancreatic tissue. There is tissue necrosis and severe inflammation of pancreas. Leakage of enzymes into general circulation may cause shock, disseminated intravascular coagulation, and acute respiratory distress syndrome. Leakage of enzymes into the peritoneal cavity continues to destroy tissue and cause massive inflammation, leading to: severe pain, hemorrhage and shock, peritonitis, and hypovolemic shock.

43. (p. 469) Manifestations include severe epigastric or abdominal pain radiating to the back; increases when supine; signs of shock: low blood pressure, pallor, and sweating; rapid but weak pulse, low-grade fever; and abdominal distention and decreased bowel sounds.

44. (p. 469) Treatment includes stopping all oral intake; relieving bowel distention; treating shock and electrolyte imbalances; and prescribing analgesics but NOT morphine.

45. (p. 470) malabsorption syndrome, primarily in childhood; genetic factors resulting in defect in intestinal enzymes needed to complete digestion of gliadin, a breakdown product of gluten

46. (p. 470, Fig. 20-29B) The combination of a digestive block with an immunologic response results in a toxic effect on the intestinal villi; villi atrophy result-

ing in decreased enzyme production and reduced surface area for absorption of nutrients, resulting in malabsorption and malnutrition

47. (p. 470) Steatorrhea, muscle wasting, and failure to gain weight; irritability and malaise are common.

48. (p. 471) Treatment is adopting a gluten-free diet, avoiding grains such as wheat, barley, and oats.

49. (p. 474, Fig. 20-32, p. 475)

obstruction of the appendiceal lumen by a fecalith, gallstone, or foreign material or from twisting or spasm

fluid builds up inside the appendix and pathogens proliferate

inflammation with purulent exudate; appendix swells, compressing blood vessels

increasing pressure and congestion leads to ischemia and necrosis, resulting in increased permeability of the wall

bacteria and toxins escape through the wall into the area; abscess formation or localized bacterial peritonitis

abscess develops when adjacent omentum adheres to appendiceal surface in an attempt to wall off the inflammation

localized infection or peritonitis develop and may spread along peritoneal membranes

necrosis and gangrene develop in the appendiceal wall

the appendix ruptures or perforates, releasing contents into the peritoneal cavity

50. (pp. 474-475)

general periumbilical pain

nausea and vomiting

increasing severity of pain, which becomes localized in lower right quadrant (LRQ)

LRQ tenderness

pain may subside temporarily with rupture

pain recurs with steady, severe abdominal pain

low-grade fever and leukocytosis

onset of peritonitis include rigid abdomen, tachycardia, and hypotension

51. (p. 471) Crohn's disease and ulcerative colitis are chronic inflammatory bowel diseases of unknown etiology.

52. (pp. 471-474, Table 20-7, Fig. 20-30)

	Crohn's Disease	Ulcerative Colitis
Individuals at high risk	Whites, Ashkenazi Jews	Whites, Ashkenazi Jews, young adults (20s and 30s)
Etiology	Genetic basis; high familial tendency	Genetic basis; high familial tendency
Location of lesions	Terminal ileum; sometimes colon	Colon, rectum
Characteristics of lesions	Transmural: all layers "Skip" lesions Granuloma	Mucosa only: continuous Ulcerations
Complications	Malabsorption; malnutrition Steatorrhea Adhesions; strictures Intestinal obstruction Fistulas and fissures	Malabsorption (rarely) Toxic megacolon → obstruction Iron deficient anemia
Manifestations	Loose or semiformed stool Melena Cramping, abdominal pain Anorexia, weight loss, fatigue Delayed growth in children	Frequent watery stools with blood and mucus Cramping pain Fever Weight loss

53. (pp. 473-474) Treatment includes identification and removal of stressors, anti-inflammatory medications, antimotility agents, nutritional supplements, antimicrobials, immunotherapeutic agents, and surgical resection (ileostomy or colostomy).

54. (p. 476) A diverticulum is a herniation or outpouching of the mucosa through the muscular layer of the colon. Diverticulitis refers to inflammation of the diverticula.

55. (Fig. 20-36, p. 479) Warning signs vary depending on location of the tumor within the bowel

ascending colon: liquid stool; occult blood or melena; anemia, fatigue; late palpable mass

transverse colon: semisolid stool; anemia, occult blood, change in bowel habits

descending colon: solid stool; constipation, discomfort; abdominal fullness and distention; red or dark blood in stool

rectum: solid stool; abdominal discomfort and cramps; ribbon or pellet stool; incomplete emptying; red blood on surface of stool

56. (p. 480, Fig. 20-38) mechanical: resulting from tumors, adhesions, hernias, or other tangible obstruc-

tions; functional: adynamic obstruction due to neurologic impairment such as spinal cord injury or lack of propulsion in the intestine (*paralytic ileus*)

57. (pp. 480, 482, Fig. 20-39, p. 482) Intestinal obstruction is a mechanical obstruction of the flow of the intestinal contents. Gases and fluids accumulate in the proximal area, distending the intestine. Increasingly strong contractions occur. Increasing intraluminal pressure leads to more secretions and compression of the veins, preventing absorption. Intestinal distention leads to persistent vomiting and loss of fluid and electrolytes resulting in hypovolemia. If the obstruction is not removed, ischemia and necrosis of the intestinal wall may result leading to potential gangrene, depending on the cause. There is decreased innervation and cessation of peristalsis (decrease in bowel sounds). There is rapid overgrowth of intestinal bacteria and production of endotoxins, which leak into peritoneal cavity (peritonitis) and the bloodstream (septicemia and bacteremia). In time, there is perforation and generalized peritonitis. If the obstruction is functional rather than mechanical, then peristalsis ceases, and there is distention of intestine. There are no reflex spasms. The rest of sequence is the same as above.

58. (pp. 483-484) Manifestations include
mechanical obstruction of small intestine
 severe, colicky abdominal pain
 borborygmi (audible rumbling sounds) and intestinal rushes
 vomiting and abdominal distention occur quickly
 restlessness and sweating with tachycardia
 signs of dehydration, weakness, confusion, and shock
in paralytic ileus, bowel sounds decrease or are absent and pain is steady
large intestine obstruction: develops slowly and signs are mild
 constipation and mild lower abdominal pain
 abdominal distention, anorexia
 vomiting and more severe pain

59. (p. 484) inflammation of the peritoneal membranes

60. (p. 484) chemical irritation; bacterial invasion

61. (pp. 484-485, Fig. 20-41)
local inflammation of the peritoneum and omentum producing a thick, sticky exudate; abscess formation; reduction in peristalsis (attempts to keep inflammation; infection localized)
rapid dissemination of irritants or bacteria throughout abdomen with distention and reflex abdominal spasm (involvement of parietal peritoneum)
vasodilation and increased capillary permeability of peritoneal membrane; edema; leakage of fluid into peritoneal cavity ("third spacing"); hypovolemic shock
fluid becomes sequestered in peritoneal cavity; leaked fluid becomes purulent as infection spreads; nausea and vomiting from intestinal irritation and pain, adding to fluid/electrolyte loss
complications if intervention delayed; nerve conduc-

tion is impaired, peristalsis decreases leading to obstruction; movement of bacteria and toxins into bloodstream resulting in bacteremia and septicemia

62. (p. 485) Manifestations include sudden and severe generalized abdominal pain, localized tenderness, pain increasing with movement (individual often restricts breathing), vomiting, signs of dehydration and hypovolemia, fever and leukocytosis, abdominal distention, rigid abdomen (involvement of parietal peritoneum), and decreased bowel sound (paralytic ileus and secondary obstruction).

63. (p. 485) Interventions include surgery and drainage of infection site, antimicrobial drugs, replacement therapy, and nasogastric suction to relieve distention.

64. (pp. 436-438, Table 20-3)
 i. prednisone: anti-inflammatory; e.g., inflammatory bowel disease (Crohn's, ulcerative colitis)
 ii. dimenhydrinate: antiemetic; e.g., acute gastritis, gastroenteritis
 iii. clarithromycin: antibiotic; e.g., peptic ulcers, inflammatory bowel disease (Crohn's, ulcerative colitis), diverticular disease, peritonitis
 iv. ranitidine: acid reduction—proton pump inhibitor; e.g., hiatus hernia, gastroesophageal reflux disease, chronic gastritis
 v. loperamide: antidiarrheal; e.g., gastroenteritis, dumping syndrome, inflammatory bowel disease (Crohn's, ulcerative colitis)
 vi. psyllium: laxative; e.g., diverticular disease
 vii. sucralfate: coating agent; e.g., chronic gastritis, gastroesophageal reflux disease, peptic ulcer

CHAPTER 21

Urinary System Disorders

1. (pp. 502-503, Fig. 21-6) Hemodialysis is provided in a hospital or dialysis center. A patient's blood moves via an implanted shunt through a dialysis machine, where exchange of wastes, fluid, and electrolytes takes place across a semipermeable membrane via ultrafiltration, diffusion, and osmosis and then is returned to the patient's bloodstream. Peritoneal dialysis is administered at home or in a dialysis unit and can be administered while patient is asleep or ambulatory. Dialyzing fluid is instilled via catheter into the peritoneal cavity and allowed to remain there, facilitating exchanges of wastes and electrolytes by diffusion and osmosis across a semipermeable membrane; then the dialysate is drained from the cavity via gravity into a container.

2. (p. 502) Complications include an infected shunt or formation of blood clots, sclerosis and damage to blood vessels involved in the shunt, and increased risk of infection by hepatitis virus or HIV.

3. (Think About, p. 502) Although rare, there is always the possibility that the equipment was not sterilized properly and the dialysis patient will be exposed to these viruses.

4. (p. 504) Any invasive procedure such as dental scaling or extractions may introduce bacteria into the blood, resulting in a temporary bacteremia.

5. (pp. 504-505, Fig. 21-7) Predisposing factors include prostatic hypertrophy and urinary retention in older men, congenital abnormalities in children, incomplete bladder emptying, reduced fluid intake, impaired blood supply to the bladder, and immobility. Women are anatomically more vulnerable to infection because of the shortness and width of the urethra, its proximity to the anus; and the frequent irritation to the tissues caused by sexual activity, tampons, bubble bath, and deodorants.

6. (pp. 509-510) Manifestations of cystitis include lower abdominal pain; dysuria, urgency, frequency, and nocturia; systemic signs of infection (fever, malaise, nausea, and leukocytosis); cloudy urine with an unusual odor; and urinalysis indicating bacteriuria. Manifestations of pyelonephritis include signs and symptoms of cystitis, pain associated with renal disease (dull aching pain in lower back), more marked systemic signs, and urinalysis similar to that of cystitis plus the addition of urinary casts.

7. (p. 507, Figs. 21-9, 21-10) Antistreptococcal antibodies, resulting from earlier infection, create an antigen-antibody complex that lodges in the glomerular capillaries, activating the complement to cause an inflammatory response in both kidneys. This leads to increased capillary permeability and cell proliferation, resulting in leakage of protein and RBCs into the glomerular filtrate. When inflammation is severe, it interferes with filtration, causing decreased GFR and fluid retention. Acute renal failure is possible if blood flow is sufficiently impaired. Renin secretion is likely to be triggered, leading to elevated blood pressure and edema. If the process becomes chronic, the kidneys are scarred.

8. (p. 507) Manifestations include
   dark and cloudy urine
   facial and periorbital edema, followed by generalized edema
   elevated blood pressure
   flank pain
   general signs of inflammation, including malaise, fatigue, headache, anorexia, and nausea
   oliguria

9. (p. 507)
   blood tests showing elevated serum urea and creatinine, elevated antistreptococcal antibodies (ASO and ASK), and decreased complement level
   metabolic acidosis with low serum pH and bicarbonate
   proteinuria, gross hematuria, and erythrocyte casts

10. (p. 509)
    abnormality in the glomerular capillaries and increased permeability resulting in proteinuria (albuminuria)
    hypoalbuminemia leading to generalized edema due to decreased plasma osmotic pressure
    low or normal blood pressure with hypovolemia or elevated depending on angiotensin levels
    hypovolemia leading to aldosterone secretion and more severe edema
    high levels of blood cholesterol and lipoprotein in the urine due to unknown factors, possibly liver response to protein loss in the urine

11. (p. 509) Most significant manifestation: massive edema or anasarca
    potential consequences include:
    weight gain
    pallor
    anorexia
    dyspnea
    decreased exercise tolerance
    skin breakdown and subsequent infection

12. (p. 509) glucocorticoids, ACE inhibitors, and antihypertensives

13. (pp. 510-511) Causative factors include excessive amounts of insoluble salts in the filtrate, e.g., hypercalcemia due to hyperparathyroidism; hyperuricemia due to gout or cancer chemotherapy

14. (p. 511) Small stones that are "passed" will be visible and can be analyzed for content.

15. (p. 511) Manifestations include flank pain due to distention of the renal capsule, renal colic (intense spasms of pain in the flank area radiating into the groin), perhaps accompanied by nausea and vomiting, cool moist skin, and rapid pulse; confirmed by radiologic examination.

16. (p. 511) buildup of urine due to obstruction of outflow, causing a dilated area proximal to the obstruction in either ureter or kidney and resulting in tissue atrophy and necrosis

17. (p. 511, Fig. 21-11, p. 510) secondary complication of: calculi, tumors, scar tissue in the kidney or ureter, stenosis or kinking of the ureter and untreated prostatic enlargement; developmental defects

18. (p. 512) "arteriosclerosis" of renal vasculature

19. (p. 512) primary vascular changes in the kidney or secondary to essential hypertension, diabetes mellitus (see diabetic nephropathy and Fig. 25-5 in Chapter 25), or another condition

20. (pp. 514-517, Fig. 21-15, Table 21-3) Causes include nephrotoxins; ischemia; and pyelonephritis.

21. (p. 516) Reverse the primary problem quickly and provide dialysis.

22. (pp. 516-517, Table 21-3) Causes include nephrosclerosis, diabetes mellitus, nephrotoxins, chronic exposure, chronic bilateral kidney inflammation or infection, and polycystic disease.

23. (pp. 516-517, Fig. 21-16) Renal insufficiency is the second stage of chronic renal failure when about 75% of the nephrons are lost. End-stage renal failure or uremia occurs when more than 90% of nephrons are lost and GFR is negligible.

24. (pp. 516, 518, Table 21-3, Fig. 21-16):
    i. fluid and electrolyte balance: fluid, wastes retained; all body systems affected; oliguria

or anuria; hypocalcemia, hyperphosphatemia, hyponatremia, hyperkalemia; acidosis

  ii. cardiovascular: CHF, arrhythmias, hypertension

  iii. central nervous system: encephalopathy (lethargy, memory lapses, seizures, tremors)

  iv. musculoskeletal: osteodystrophy (Fig. 21-17, p. 518), osteoporosis, and tetany

  v. endocrine: impotence and decreased libido in men; menstrual irregularities in women

  vi. skin and mucosa: dry, pruritic and hyperpigmented skin; easy bruising; uremic frost in terminal stage

25. (pp. 516-518)

  i. metabolic acidosis: GFR declines and tubule function is lost

  ii. hyperkalemia: potassium retained as GFR decreases

  iii. hypocalcemia: decreased renal activation of vitamin D leading to decreased GI calcium absorption; high phosphate levels

  iv. increased serum urea and serum creatinine: decreased GFR

  v. anemia: decreased production of erythropoietin leading to decreased RBC production; bone marrow depression

  vi. delayed clotting: red bone marrow function depressed by altered blood chemistry that leads to decreased platelet production

  vii. edema: increased blood volume due to decreased GFR

  viii. increased blood pressure: increased blood volume; increased renin secretion

  ix. cardiac arrhythmias: electrolyte imbalances, particularly hypocalcemia and hyperkalemia

  x. congestive heart failure: increased blood volume and increased blood pressure

  xi. pulmonary edema: due to development of heart failure

  xii. lethargy, confusion: due to accumulation of nitrogenous wastes in blood, particularly urea: acidosis

  xiii. muscle weakness: due to hypocalcemia and encephalopathy

  xiv. bone tenderness: due to bone demineralization (hypocalcemia stimulates secretion of PTH, which causes bone resorption)

  xv. amenorrhea: abnormal metabolism of hormones; increased wastes in serum

  xvi. severe pruritis: due to presence of uremic frost

  xvii. ammonia smelling breath: urea catabolism; ammonia being excreted in respirations

  xviii. hypoplasia of tooth enamel: due to hypocalcemia with resulting in increased secretion of PTH

26. (Think About, p. 519)

Most drugs are excreted primarily via the kidney. With renal failure, the rate of drug excretion decreases, resulting in accumulation of the medication. This can result in increased adverse, potentially toxic drug effects.

27. answer to crossword puzzle

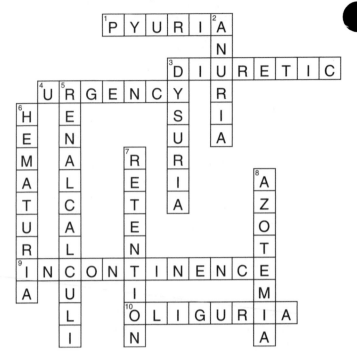

CHAPTER 22

Acute Neurologic Disorders

1. (pp. 541-542, Fig. 22-6) brain hemorrhage, trauma, cerebral edema, infection, tumors, or accumulation of excessive amounts of cerebrospinal fluid (CSF)

2. (pp. 540, Table 22-7)
increase in pressure in the brain
decrease in arterial blood flood into the "high pressure" area
pressure increases at the site of the problem initially but gradually is dispersed throughout the CNS
brain compression
decrease functionality of neurons, both locally and generally
brain death

3. (pp. 541-543, Table 22-7)
Early manifestations:
decreasing level of consciousness or responsiveness (lethargy); pressure on RAS (brainstem) or cerebral cortex
severe headache; stretching or distortion of meninges or walls of large blood vessels
vomiting; Pressure on emetic center in medulla
increasing blood pressure with increasing pulse pressure; Cushing's reflex, response to cerebral ischemia causes systemic vasoconstriction
slow heart rate; response to increasing blood pressure
papilledema; increased pressure of CSF causes swelling around the optic disc
pupil becomes fixed and dilated on ipsilateral side of lesion initially, eventually, both pupils become

fixed and dilated; Pressure on cranial nerve III (oculomotor)

4. (p. 544) Signs of increased intracranial pressure, often beginning with morning headaches that increase in severity and frequency; vomiting; and lethargy and irritability; focal or generalized seizures may be the first sign.

5. (p. 546) temporary localized reduction of blood flow in the brain

6. (p. 546) The manifestations of TIA are directly related to the location of the ischemia. The patient remains conscious. Intermittent short episodes of impaired function, such as muscle weakness in an arm or leg, visual disturbances, or numbness and paresthesia in the face, may occur. Transient aphasia or confusion may develop. The attack may last a few minutes or longer but rarely lasts more than 1 to 2 hours, and then the signs disappear.

7. (p. 546) They warn of the potential development of an obstruction leading to a cerebrovascular event.

8. (p. 546) TIAs do not cause permanent brain damage; a CVA does. TIAs are caused by partial arterial obstruction or spasm; CVAs are caused by total obstruction or hemorrhage.

9. (p. 547) Individuals with
diabetes
hypertension, especially if chronic, severe in the elderly
systemic lupus erythematosus
hypercholesterolemia
atherosclerosis

history of TIAs
increasing age
heart disease
combination of oral contraceptives and cigarette smoking

10. (Warning Signs box, p. 548)
sudden transient weakness, numbness, or tingling in the face, an arm or leg, or on one side
temporary loss of speech, failure to comprehend, or contusion
sudden loss of vision
sudden severe headache
unusual dizziness or unsteadiness

11. (p. 546)
occlusion of an artery by an atheroma (most common)
embolism lodging in the cerebral artery
intracerebral hemorrhage

12. (pp. 546-547, Fig. 22-11) Infarction of brain tissue results from lack of blood; tissue necrosis results from total occlusion of a cerebral blood vessel or the consequence of a ruptured cerebral vessel. Within 5 minutes of ischemia, irreversible cell damage occurs. A central area of necrosis develops, surrounded by an area of inflammation. With time the tissue liquefies, leaving a cavity. The cerebral edema increases the neurological deficits. As the edema decreases, functions performed by the inflamed area start to return.

13. (pp. 546-548, Table 22-8)

	Thrombus CVA	Embolus CVA	Hemorrhage CVA
Predisposing factors	Atherosclerosis	Atherosclerosis Rheumatic heart disease Valvular disease Prosthetic heart valves Endocarditis Arrhythmias Heart failure	Hypertension
Onset	Gradual May be preceded by TIAs Often at rest	Sudden	Sudden
Effects	Localized	Localized	Widespread Increased ICP Often fatal
Immediate treatment	Fibrinolytic agents— "clot buster" Thrombectomy O$_2$	Fibrinolytic agents Thrombectomy	Ligation of ruptured vessel if accessible
Prognosis	Depends on size and location of injury, plus speed of initiation of treatment	Depends on size and location of injury, plus speed of initiation of treatment	Depends on size and location of injury, plus speed of initiation of treatment Worst prognosis—most often fatal

14. (p. 546)

left side of heart: rheumatic heart disease, endo-carditis, valvular disease, prosthetic heart valves, left-sided heart failure, arrhythmias

carotid arteries

15. (pp. 546-547)

because damage much more widespread—often increased ICP

both hemispheres involved

sudden onset—no time for development of collateral circulation

secondary effects of bleeding: vasospasm, electrolyte imbalances, acidosis, cellular edema

16. (p. 548, Fig. 22-1, p. 526) Signs and symptoms depend on location of the obstruction, size of artery involved, and the functional area affected. However, the four general types of deficits include:

i. motor deficits: contralateral muscle weakness or paralysis (hemiplegia)

ii. sensory deficits: contralateral paresthesia or numbness; possibly loss of vision

iii. speech: aphasia when the dominant side of the brain is involved

iv. cognitive and emotional: confusion, loss of problem-solving skills, personality changes, impairment of spatial relationships

17. (pp. 548-549)

medications: depend on underlying problem
antihypertensives
platelet inhibitors or anticoagulants
laxatives
physiotherapy
occupational therapy
speech therapy

18. (p. 548, Fig. 22-1, p. 526) loss of movement and sensation on the right side of the body (contralateral); expressive or motor aphasia

19. (p. 549) localized dilation in an artery

20. (p. 550) increased blood pressure, for example, during exertion

21. (p. 550) Enlarging aneurysm may cause pressure on the surrounding structures, such as the optic chiasm or cranial nerves, resulting in vision disturbances and headaches as tension increases on the vessel wall and meninges. Small leaks cause headaches, photophobia, and periods of confusion, slurred speech, or weakness. Nuchal rigidity may develop. Massive ruptures result in immediate severe headaches, vomiting, photophobia, and perhaps seizures or loss of consciousness. Death may occur shortly after rupture.

22. (pp. 550-553)

	Meningitis	Encephalitis
Causative agents	Meningococci *Escherichia coli* Influenza Pneumococci	Western equine virus West Nile virus Herpes simplex
Predisposing factors	Other infections (sinusitis, otitis, mumps, measles) Abscessed tooth Head trauma or surgery	Insect bites
Pathophysiology	Increased ICP Edema of arachnoid and pia maters Purulent exudates that cover brain surface and is in CSF	Infection involves parenchyma of brain and cord, especially basal ganglia May include meninges Necrosis and inflammation may lead to permanent damage
Manifestations	Sudden onset Severe headache, back pain, photophobia Nuchal rigidity Vomiting Irritability, lethargy, stupor, or seizures Fever and chills Leukocytosis	Severe headache Stiff neck Vomiting Lethargy Seizures Fever
Treatment	Appropriate antimicrobial agent	Antiviral agent if available Supportive measures

23. (pp. 555-556, Fig. 22-15)
    i. base of the skull
    ii. bleeding between the dura mater and the cranium
    iii. bleeding between the dural and arachnoid maters
    iv. bleeding into the space between the arachnoid and pia maters, where CSF is located
    v. bleeding within the brain
24. (pp. 555-558, Figs. 22-15, 22-16)
    skull fracture: tissue damage and bleeding resulting in increased ICP, ischemia and necrosis; compression of brain stem with potential loss of vital functions

    contusion: edema and minor bleeding

    brain motion: tissue damage and bleeding resulting in increased ICP, ischemia and necrosis; compression of brain stem with potential loss of vital functions

    secondary damage due to bleeding, inflammation and edema; hematoma and possible infection; tissue damage and bleeding resulting in increased ICP, ischemia and necrosis; compression of brain stem with potential loss of vital functions

    if unconscious for a prolonged period, other problems may develop; immobility may result in pneumonia or decubitus ulcers (p. 559)
25. (pp. 558-559)
    seizures (see Chapter 23)

    cranial nerve impairment

    otorrhea or rhinorrhea—leaking of CSF from the ear or nose, respectively

    otorrhagia—blood leaking from the ear

    fever due to hypothalamic impairment or of cranial or systemic infection

    stress ulcers—from increased gastric secretions
26. (p. 560) glucocorticoids, antimicrobials, surgery, oxygen therapy
27. (p. 560; Fig. 22-19, p. 561)
    hyperextension or hyperflexion of the neck

    dislocation of vertebra

    compression fractures

    penetrating injuries such as stab or bullet wounds

    decreased responses
28. (pp. 560-565; Figs. 22-19, 22-21, 22-22)
    Damage may be temporary or permanent; laceration of nerve tissue usually results in permanent loss of conduction in affected nerve tracts.

    Complete transection or crushing causes irreversible loss of all function at and below the level of injury.

Partial transection may allow recovery of some function.

Bruising is reversible damage when edema and bleeding are mild.

Prolonged ischemia and necrosis lead to permanent damage.

Edema and hemorrhage occur above and below the injury.

Impaired respiration may occur when injury occurs in cervical region.

Spinal shock can occur.

Complications are due to autonomic dysreflexia, immobility, contractures and decubitus ulcers, respiratory and urinary infections, loss of function, e.g. sexual function and reproductive capacity affected.

29. (pp. 563-565, Fig. 22-21) Manifestations depend on the level of the cord at which the injury occurred as well as the time that has elapsed since the injury (i.e., early stage of spinal shock or postspinal shock).

    spinal shock (immediately following injury)
        all function normal above the level of inflammation
        no sensory or motor impulses below the injury
        no reflexes: flaccid paralysis, no sensation, urinary retention, paralytic ileus
        low, labile blood pressure
    permanent effects—post spinal shock
        cervical injury—total block
            no sensation
            no voluntary movement (spastic paralysis)
            no central control of SNS
            no voluntary control of bladder and bowel
        lumbar injury
            normal function upper body
            no function at level of injury
            no sensory of voluntary movement below injury
            reflexes present below injury
                spastic paralysis
                bowel and bladder incontinence
30. (p. 565)
    traction or surgery to relieve pressure and repair tissues

    glucocorticoids

    supportive care and rehabilitation to prevent complications related to immobility

31. answer to crossword puzzle

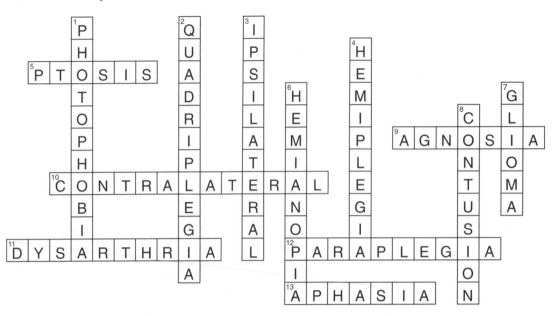

CHAPTER 23

Chronic Neurologic Disorders

1. (p. 572) a condition in which excess cerebrospinal fluid accumulates in the skull, compressing the brain tissue and blood vessels

2. (p. 572) developmental abnormalities such as stenosis or atresia; tumors, infection, or scar tissue at any age

3. (p. 572) Compression of brain tissue and blood vessels leads to brain damage; the amount and severity depend on the rate at which the pressure is increasing and the time that elapses before initiation of treatment. In severe cases, hydrocephalus can cause major physical disabilities and intellectual impairment.

4. (p. 572, Fig. 23-1) Noncommunicating or obstructive hydrocephalus occurs in babies when the flow of CSF through the ventricular system is blocked. In communicating hydrocephalus, absorption of CSF through subarachnoid villi is impaired, resulting in increased CSF pressure.

5. (p. 573) It depends on the age of the patient. In neonates or young infants (prior to suture closure), manifestations include enlarged head, bulging fontanels, dilated scalp veins, eyes showing "sunset" sign, sluggish pupil response, lethargy and restlessness, and shrill cries when infants are picked up. In older children and adults, manifestations include classic signs of increased intracranial pressure.

6. (p. 573) Treatment is surgery to remove the obstruction or provide a shunt for CSF.

7. (p. 573) neural tube defect due to failure of the vertebral posterior spinous processs to fuse

8. (pp. 573-574, Fig. 23-2)
   spina bifida occulta: develops when the spinous processes do not fuse, but herniation of the spinal cord and meninges does not occur; may not be visible; often a dimple or tuft of hair is present

   meningocele: same bony defect as spina bifida except herniation of the meninges occurs through the defect, and the meninges and CSF form a sac on the surface

   myelomeningocele: most serious form; herniation of the spinal cord and nerves along with the meninges and CSF occurs, resulting in considerable neurologic impairment; often seen in conjunction with hydrocephalus

9. (p. 574) elevated alpha-fetoprotein (AFP) in maternal blood; AFP in amniotic fluid by amniocentesis

10. (p. 574)
    multifactorial basis with both genetic and environmental factors contributing

    high familial incidence and associated defects such as anencephaly

    environmental factors include exposure to radiation, gestational diabetes, and deficits of vitamin A or folic acid

11. (p. 574)
    meningocele and myelomeningocele are visible as protrusions over the spine

    extent of neurological defect depending on level of the defect (myelomeningocele)

    impaired sensory and motor function at and below the level of herniation

    muscle weakness or paralysis

    fecal and urinary incontinence, depending on the level of damage

12. (p. 574) surgery and therapy to manage the neurologic deficits

13. (p. 575) Major causes of cerebral palsy: hypoxia or ischemia, which can occur prenatally (caused by

placental complications), perinatally (a difficult delivery), or postnatally (vascular occlusion, hemorrhage, aspiration, or respiratory impairment in the premature infant. An infection or metabolic abnormalities such as hypoglycemia in mother or infant may also cause cerebral palsy.

14. (p. 575) Necrosis of brain tissue in the perinatal period as a result of malformation, mechanical trauma, hypoxia, hemorrhage, hypoglycemia, hyperbilirubinemia; necrosis, and atrophy may be generalized or localized; all children have altered mobility and an assortment of other individual problems based on the extent of brain damage.

15. (pp. 575-576, Table 23-1)

spastic paralysis due to damage to the pyramidal tracts (diplegia), the motor cortex (hemiparesis), or general cortical damage (quadriparesis); characterized by paralysis, hyperreflexia, and increased muscle tone

dyskinetic disease due to damage to the extrapyramidal tract, basal nuclei, or cranial nerves; manifested by athetoid or choreiform involuntary movements and loss of coordination with fine movements

ataxic cerebral palsy from damage to the cerebellum and manifesting as loss of balance and coordination

16. (p. 576) impairment of intellectual function; communication and speech difficulties; seizures; visual problems

17. (p. 576)

early stimulation programs for motor skills, coordination, and intellectual development

speech and language pathology assessment to assist in feeding and swallowing problems

regular physical therapy and use of devices such as braces to improve mobility and decrease deformities

development and maximization of motor skills, eye-hand coordination and reflex responses

monitoring hearing and vision and appropriate communication therapy

medications to control seizures

18. (p. 577) an abnormal motor or sensory activity and possible loss of consciousness due to sudden, spontaneous, uncontrolled depolarization of neurons in the brain

19. (p. 577) hyperexcitable neurons in an epileptogenic focus in the brain that have a lowered threshold for stimulation and respond to a variety of stimuli with sudden, spontaneous, uncontrolled depolarization

20. (p. 578) Primary seizures are idiopathic. Secondary (acquired) seizures have an identifiable cause such as fever, drug withdrawal, or post head injury or infection

21. (p. 578) initiated by tumor, infection, or hemorrhage in the brain, high fever, and some systemic disorders (renal failure or hypoglycemia) or sudden withdrawal from sedatives or alcohol or narcotics

22. (Box 23-1, p. 577)

generalized seizure: has multiple foci in deep structures of both cerebral hemispheres and the brainstem—causes loss of consciousness

partial seizure: single origin, often in cerebral cortex —may or may not cause altered consciousness

23. (p. 578) An absence or petit mal seizure is a generalized seizure that is more common in children, lasts for 5 to 10 seconds, and may occur many times during the day. There is a brief loss of awareness (child may simply stare into space) and sometimes transient facial movements, which may occur several times a day, with no memory of the episode.

24. (p. 578) In some individuals, signs such as nausea, irritability, depression, or muscle twitching may occur some hours before the onset of a seizure.

25. (p. 578) Peculiar visual or auditory or olfactory sensation that immediately precedes the loss of consciousness; examples of auras are the smell of burnt toast, bright flashing lights, buzzing sounds; the significance of an aura is that a seizure is imminent.

26. (p. 578) physical stimuli such as loud noises or bright lights; biochemical stimuli such as stress, excessive premenstrual fluid retention, hypoglycemia, or hyperventilation (alkalosis)

27. (p. 578) A tonic-clonic seizure may occur spontaneously or after simple seizures. The pattern for this type of seizure is:

tonic stage:

- nausea, irritability, depression, or muscle twitching
- aura (which may precede a loss of consciousness in some persons)
- loss of consciousness
- strong tonic muscle contraction
- jaws clench, air is forced out of the lungs, a cry escapes, respiration ceases

clonic stage:

- muscles contract and relax in a series of jerky movements involving the entire body
- increased salivation (foaming at the mouth), bowel/bladder incontinence may occur
- contractions subside, the body turns limp, and consciousness eventually returns
- person is confused and tired, muscles ache, falls into deep sleep

typical duration is several minutes, shouldn't last longer than 5 minutes

28. (p. 579) hypoxia, airway obstruction, acidosis, status epilepticus, cuts and lacerations of tongue and oral mucosa sustained during seizure, broken teeth from falling

29. (Emergency Treatment box, p. 579)

30. (Think About, p. 580)

if individual stopped breathing during seizure

when a seizure lasts more than 5 minutes

when one seizure immediately follows another

if individual hurts himself (e.g., due to fall at onset of seizure)

if individual has not recovered consciousness after 30 minutes

31. (Box 23-1, p. 577)

simple partial seizure: arises from a single damaged area, often in cortex

- characterized by repeated motor activity

211

- memory and consciousness remain

complex partial seizure: usually arises from temporal lobe with possible limbic system or frontal lobe involvement
- characterized by bizarre behavior that may be mistaken for psychiatric condition, such as inappropriate repetitive movements
- frequently experiences auditor or visual hallucinations
- individual is unresponsive

32. (pp. 579-580) anticonvulsants and barbiturates

33. (pp. 579-580) Adverse effects of anticonvulsants include leukopenia with increased susceptibility to infection and reduced blood clotting ability and gingival hyperplasia (particularly phenytoin).

Adverse effects of barbiturates include increased liver enzyme activity affecting the dosage of other medications, drowsiness, and osteomalacia.

34. (pp. 579, 580) Status epilepticus are recurrent tonic-clonic seizures without return to full consciousness. They can be life-threatening. IV diazepam, oxygen, and fluids are used to treat this condition.

35. (Think About, pp. 578-579)

How well is the individual's disorder controlled—when was the last seizure and how frequently do they occur?

known precipitating factors: stress, bright lights, certain noises or odors, hyperventilation, exercise, hot environmental temperatures, recent alcohol consumption, nitrous oxide

presence of an "aura": What are the signs of an impending seizure, and how much time between the aura and the onset of a seizure?

How long do seizures usually last?

How long does it take to recover from a seizure?

What does the individual want you to do if he has a seizure (e.g., who to notify)?

36. (p. 578) awareness and avoidance of potential precipitating factors; stress reduction, which may require sedation (e.g., prior to a dental treatment)

37. (p. 581) unknown etiology; possibly autoimmune disorder with genetic, immunologic, and environmental components

38. (p. 581) women between the ages of 20 and 40; individuals of European descent; those living in temperate climates; close relatives of individuals with MS

39. (p. 580, Fig. 23-7, p. 581) Progressive diffuse demyelination of the neurons of the brain, spinal cord, and cranial nerves; plaque is the characteristic lesion of MS and refers to the areas of inflammation and demyelination.

40. (p. 580) Motor, sensory, and autonomic

41. (p. 582) There is no definitive test for MS. Multiplicity of effects and recurrences based on patient history and physical examination point to the correct diagnosis. MRIs are best to detect multiple CNS lesions. Often patients have elevated protein, gamma globulin, and lymphocytes in the CSF.

42. (pp. 581-582) Early manifestations include blurred vision, weakness in the legs, scotoma, diplopia, dysarthria if the cranial nerves are involved, and paresthesias if sensory nerves affected. Progressive signs are weakness and paralysis extending to upper limbs, loss of coordination and bladder, bowel, and sexual dysfunction. Chronic fatigue and sensory deficits such as paresthesias and loss of position sense in upper body are also progressive signs. Depression or euphoria may occur later.

43. (p. 582) There is no specific treatment available. The following may be used to control exacerbations:
glucocorticoids
interferons
muscle relaxants
avoidance of excessive fatigue, stress, injury, or infection
physical therapy and exercise
specific therapies for vision, speech, etc.

44. (p. 582) Glucocorticoids will decrease inflammation and hopefully neural function will return. Interferon will suppress the immune response and hopefully slow progression of the disease.

45. (p. 582) There is progressive degenerative changes in the basal nuclei, principally in the substantia nigra. Decreased secretion of dopamine results in an imbalance between excitation and inhibition in the basal nuclei, which causes resting tremors, muscular rigidity, difficulty in initiating movement, and postural instability.

46. (pp. 582-583, Fig. 23-8) Early manifestations include fatigue, muscle weakness, muscle aching, decreased flexibility and less spontaneous change in facial expression; tremors in the hands at rest and "pill-rolling" motion. Progressive signs include tremors affecting hands, feet, face, tongue, and lips; increased muscle rigidity, difficulty in initiating movement; bradykinesia and lack of associative involuntary movements; and characteristic stooped posture. Late signs include festination or a propulsive gait; complex activities become difficult; voice changes; difficulty chewing and swallowing; drooling; mask-like facies; and autonomic dysfunction such as urinary retention, constipation, and orthostatic hypotension.

47. (p. 582) phenothiazines

48. (p. 583)
dopamine
levodopa
selegiline
anticholinergic drugs

49. (pp. 584-586)

	Amyotrophic Lateral Sclerosis	Myasthenia Gravis	Huntington's Disease
Etiology	Idiopathic, degenerative disorder 10% Genetic	Idiopathic Autoimmune Thymus disorders	Autosomal dominant disorder
Pathophysiology	Progressive loss of neurons in cerebral cortex, brain stem, and spinal cord in diffuse asymmetrical pattern	Development of IgG autoantibodies to acetylcholine receptors, preventing muscle stimulation Facial and ocular muscles first, then arm and trunk	Progressive brain atrophy, especially basal ganglia and frontal cortex Depletion of GABA Decreased brain levels of acetylcholine
Manifestations	Loss of fine motor coordination, usually in hands first Stumbling and falls Muscle cramping or twitching Dysarthria Finally, impaired swallowing and respiration	Diplopia; ptosis Loss of facial expression Difficulty chewing and swallowing Marked muscle fatigue and weakness in head, neck, and arms Upper respiratory infections	Rapid, jerky (choreiform) movements in arms and Intellectual impairment Progressive rigidity and akinesia, making voluntary movement difficult Progressive dementia
Treatment	No specific treatment Supportive measures Ultimately ventilator	Anticholinesterase agents Glucocorticoids Plasmapheresis to remove antibodies from blood Thymectomy if hyperplastic or tumor present	No specific treatment Supportive measures Muscle relaxants to control abnormal movements
Prognosis	Fatal HCO_3^- respiratory failure or infection	Fatal HCO_3^- respiratory failure or infection	Incurable—progressive Detection of carriers and genetic counseling

50. (pp. 586, 588)
Alzheimer's disease
cerebrovascular disease—multiple microinfarcts
Creutzfeldt-Jakob disease
AIDS

51. (p. 586)
progressive cortical atrophy
neurofibrillary tangles in the neurons and senile plaques containing beta-amyloid precursor protein
deficit in neurotransmitter acetylcholine

52. (p. 586) A specific cause is unknown; at least four defective genes on different chromosomes have been associated with the disease.

53. (p. 587) In the early stage, manifestations include gradual loss of memory and lack of concentration and an impaired ability to learn new information and to reason. There are behavioral changes such as irritability and hostility. Cognitive function, memory, and language skills decline; apathy, indifference, and confusion become marked; managing activities of daily living becomes increasingly difficult. In the later stages there is an inability to recognize family members; lack of awareness or interest in environment; incontinence and loss of functionality.

54. (p. 589) The following types of behavior may be exhibited:
positive symptoms such as delusions and bizarre behavior
negative symptoms such as flat emotions and decreased speech
disorganized though processes
delusions of false beliefs and ideas such as grandeur or power over others
poor problem-solving ability
short attention span
impaired communication
hallucinations or abnormal sensory perception
social withdrawal
personal self-care neglected

55. (p. 589) Frequently cause side effects related to excessive extrapyramidal activity (or parkinsonian signs) such as dystonia and tardive dyskinesia: involuntary muscle spasms in the face, neck, arms, or legs

56. (pp. 589-590)

selective serotonin reuptake inhibitors (SSRIs) such as Prozac

serotonin-norepinephrine reuptake inhibitors (SNRIs) such as Effexor

tricyclic antidepressants (TCAs) such as Elavil

monamine oxidase (MAO) inhibitors such as Parnate

57. (pp. 590-591; Fig. 23-11) protrusion of the nucleus pulposus, the inner gelatinous component of the intervertebral disc) through a tear in the annulus fibrosus, the outer covering of the intervertebral disc

58. (p. 591) compression of the spinal cord

59. (pp. 590-591) The most common site of a herniated disc is at the lumbosacral discs, at L4 to L5 or L5 to S1. This results in lower back pain, radiating down one or both legs, that is exacerbated by coughing or straight leg-raising. Paresthesia, or numbness and tingling, as well as muscle weakness, if compression is severe (motor nerves), may result.

60. (p. 591) conservative treatment, including bed rest; application of heat, ice, or traction, or drugs such as analgesics, anti-inflammatory agents, and skeletal muscle relaxants; surgery if compression persists: laminectomy or discectomy; chemonucleolysis; fusion

61. (Think About, (pp. 587-589)

nature of the disorder—etiology, is it progressive

duration and degree of impairment

Who is the primary care provider?

62. (Think About, (pp. 587-589)

Try to arrange for person who is responsible for care to be present at appointments.

Always provide written instructions regarding follow-up treatment, etc.—this is particularly important for individuals who are living in group homes or nursing homes where there are multiple care providers.

Provide clear explanations.

Provide demonstrations whenever possible; e.g., how to floss teeth.

63. (pp. 580-587)

   i. loss of myelin in the CNS: multiple sclerosis

   ii. impairment of receptors at neuromuscular junctions: myasthenia gravis

   iii. deterioration of basal ganglia: Parkinson's and Huntington's

   iv. development of neurofibrillary tangles: Alzheimer's

   v. decreased dopamine synthesis: Parkinson's

   vi. depletion of GABA: Huntington's

   vii. degeneration of both upper and lower motor neurons: amyotrophic lateral sclerosis (ALS)

   viii. an autosomal dominant disorder: Huntington's

   ix. an autoimmune disorder: multiple sclerosis, myasthenia gravis

   x. characterized by rigidity and difficulty initiating movements: Parkinson's

   xi. development of plaques in the brain: multiple sclerosis, Alzheimer's

   xii. decreased levels of acetylcholine in the CNS: Huntington's and Alzheimer's

   xiii. treated with levodopa: Parkinson's

   xiv. treated with donepezil: Alzheimer's

   xv. caused by infection by a prion: Creutzfeldt-Jakob disease

CHAPTER 24

Disorders of Eye and Ear

1. (pp. 601-602, Fig. 24-4) increased intraocular pressure caused by an excessive accumulation of aqueous humor

2. (pp. 601-602, Fig. 24-4) Narrow-angle glaucoma occurs when the angle between the cornea and the iris in the anterior chamber is decreased by factors such as abnormal anterior insertion of the iris. Wide-angle, or chronic, glaucoma is a degenerative disorder in older persons. The trabecular network and canal of Schlemm become obstructed, diminishing the outflow of aqueous humor

3. (p. 601) the elderly, over age 50

4. (pp. 601-602)

increased intraocular pressure

loss of peripheral vision

corneal edema and altered light refraction, leading to blurred vision and appearance of "halos" around lights

mild eye discomfort

acute episodes may be triggered by pupil dilation (narrow-angle)

eye pain, nausea, and headache; blurred vision; bulging and cloudy cornea

pupil dilated and unresponsive to light

5. (pp. 602-603) Therapeutic interventions include regular administration of β-adrenergic blockers (reduce secretions) or cholinergic agents (contract the pupil) and/or surgery, such as laser iridotomy, for acute narrow-angle glaucoma if severe.

6. (pp. 603-604)

	Cataract	Macular Degeneration	Detached Retina
Etiology	Aging Metabolic abnormalities Maternal infections	Aging Genetics Environmental factors	Marked myopia Aging Scar tissue
Pathology	Progressive clouding of lens	Growth of membrane over retina, starting at fovea centralis	Retina lifted from choroid as vitreous seeps behind tear, retinal cells stop functioning and may die
Effect on vision	Progressive blurring and darkening of vision	Loss of central vision Altered depth perception	"Floaters"—light or dark floating spots Growing area of blackness in visual field
Treatment	Lens removal and replacement with intraocular lens	Limited by type Photoactivated drugs Laser treatment	Scleral buckling Laser therapy

7. (pp. 601-604)
   i. characterized by clouding of the ocular lens: cataracts
   ii. characterized by degeneration of the fovea centralis: macular degeneration
   iii. treated with cholinergic eye drops: glaucoma
   iv. characterized by loss of central vision: macular degeneration
   v. appearances of "halos" around lights: glaucoma
   vi. increased intraocular pressure: glaucoma
8. (p. 606) Conduction deafness occurs when sound is blocked in the external or middle ear. For example, wax accumulation, a foreign object, scar tissue, or adhesions may cause conduction deafness. Sensorineural deafness is due to damage to the organ of Corti or auditory nerve. For example, infection, particularly viral, such as rubella, influenza, or herpes; head trauma; or ototoxic drugs may cause sensorineural deafness.
9. (p. 609) a disorder of the inner ear or labyrinth due to intermittent development of excessive endolymph that stretches the membranes and interferes with function of the hair cells in the cochlea and vestibule
10. (p. 609) manifestations include episodes lasting minutes or hour causing vertigo, tinnitus, and unilateral hearing loss
11. (pp. 608-609)
   i. otitis media: infants and young children
   ii. otitis externa: swimmers; frequent users of ear plugs or earphones

CHAPTER 25

Endocrine Disorders

1. (p. 618, Table 25-2) Familial history (type 1); obesity, advancing age (type 2)
2. (pp. 618-619, Table 25-2)
   Type 1
      genetic factor (family history
      autoimmune destruction of pancreatic beta cells
   Type 2
      familial, lifestyle, and environmental factors, especially obesity
3. (p. 619) An insulin deficit leads to the following sequence of events:
   decreased transportation and use of glucose
   hyperglycemia
   glucosuria
   polyuria with loss of fluid and electrolytes
   fluid loss through the urine and high blood glucose levels—dehydration
   polydipsia due to dehydration
   lack of nutrients entering the cells, stimulating appetite and leading to polyphagia
   catabolism of fats and proteins due to lack of glucose in cells; resulting in ketosis as metabolites accumulate—ketoacidosis
   ketonuria
   glomerular filtration drops, resulting in decompensated metabolic acidosis
4. (pp. 619-623, Fig. 25-4) The lack of glucose in cells results in catabolism of fats, leading to excessive buildup of fatty acids and their metabolites, ketone (ketoacids).
5. (pp. 624-625, Table 25-3) Warning signs include
   polyuria: hyperglycemia results in excess glucose in the urine as renal tubular reabsorption capacity is exceeded; the glucose in the filtrate exerts osmotic pressure, increasing the volume of urine produced
   polydipsia: fluid and electrolyte loss due to glucosuria results in dehydration and stimulation of the thirst response (hypothalamus)
   polyphagia: lack of nutrients in cells stimulates appetite
   weight loss: particularly with type 1, due to fat catabolism

6. (pp. 619-620) Diagnosis is established from the following: fasting blood glucose level, glucose tolerance test, and glycosylated hemoglobin test.

7. (p. 620) Dietary modifications include dieting to reduce weight or maintain optimum weight, adding more complex carbohydrates, adequate protein and low saturated fats and fiber to reduce cholesterol levels, minimal intake of simple and refined sugars, and balancing and reducing food intake to match insulin availability, metabolic needs, and activity level.

8. (p. 620) Oral hypoglycemics act in a number of different ways to lower blood sugar; some stimulate beta cells to release more insulin, others reduce insulin resistance of cells and hepatic glucose production, and another type increases cell sensitivity to insulin

9. (p. 618) Oral hypoglycemics are effective only if the person is still synthesizing insulin. Individuals with type 1 diabetes have absolute insulin deficiency; they are not producing any insulin.

10. (Think About)
hypoglycemia
gastrointestinal disturbances; anorexia, nausea, vomiting
anemia
pruritis (itching)
liver and kidney damage
metallic taste (with metformin)

11. (pp. 620-621) The various forms of insulin differ in onset of action, peak insulin levels, and duration of action.

12. (pp. 620-621) Insulin can be administered by subcutaneous injections, continuous subcutaneous infusion ("insulin pump"), or inhalation, which was just approved by the FDA.

13. (pp. 621-622, Fig. 26-3) Factors that could precipitate a hypoglycaemic or insulin reaction include increased physical exercise, skipping a meal or fasting, delayed or inadequate food intake, insulin overdose (too much insulin), and nutritional and/or fluid and electrolyte imbalances due to nausea and vomiting.

14. (p. 621)
Verify that patients have eaten and taken appropriate medications.
Schedule appointments that do not unduly delay meals.

15. (pp. 624-625, Table 25-4)

16. (p. 625) Diabetic neuropathy is a disorder of peripheral nerves that produces impaired sensation, numbness, tingling, weakness, and muscle wasting. It results from ischemia and altered metabolic process. Degenerative changes occur in both unmyelinated and myelinated fibers. There is a risk of tissue trauma and infection. Autonomic nerve degeneration leads to bladder incontinence, impotence, diarrhea, and impaired vasomotor reflexes. Vascular impairment decreases tissue resistance and slows healing; sensory impairment means that an individual may not realize that he has injured himself and therefore does not implement appropriate measures.

17. (p. 625) Risk of infection is greatly increased when vascular and sensory impairment coexist.

18. (pp. 625-626)
tuberculosis
infections in the feet and hands
fungal infections
urinary tract infections
periodontal disease

19. (p. 625) There may be delayed healing because of decreased circulation to injured site due to both macroangiopathy and microangiopathy. Individuals are more prone to infections, which will further delay healing. If diabetes is poorly controlled, protein synthesis will be decreased due to ongoing gluconeogenesis and protein catabolism.

20. (p. 618 and Chapter 9) diabetes that develops during pregnancy and usually ends with the delivery of the infant

21. (Think About, pp. 617-619)
What type of diabetes does the client have?
What was the age of onset? This is an indication of the duration of the disease—the longer he has had it, the more likely he is of having some of the many complications.
What is the level of blood sugar control? Does the individual monitor his own blood glucose levels? What is the average range of his blood glucose?
How often does he have a hypoglycemic reaction? When was the last one?
Does he have much warning?
What works best for him if he does have a hypoglycemic reaction?

22. (pp. 621-624; Figs. 25-3 and 25-4)

	Hypoglycemic Shock	**Ketoacidosis**
Other names	Insulin shock Insulin reaction	Diabetic coma
Cause	Hypoglycemia	Hyperglycemia

Precipitating factors	Increased physical exercise
	Skipping a meal or fasting
	Delayed or inadequate food intake
	Insulin overdose—too much insulin
	Nutritional and/or fluid and electrolyte
	    imbalances due to nausea and vomiting
		Excessive food and/or alcohol intake
		Inadequate insulin—skipped or delayed
		Increased requirement for insulin:
		    infection, stress, glucocorticoids

Speed of onset	Rapid	Slow

Manifestations	Apprehensive, headache
	Pale, cold, diaphoretic, "clammy"
	Hungry, thirsty
	Appears intoxicated: unexpected
	    behavior, slurred speech, incoherent,
	    disoriented, staggering gait
	Difficulty problem solving
	Muscle twitching, tremors
	Seizures
	Permanent brain damage
	Death
		Increased hunger and thirst
		Polyuria
		Fatigue, confusion
		Nausea and vomiting
		Signs of dehydration: flushed:
		    warm, dry skin and mucous
		    membranes
		Acetone breath
		Tachycardia and lowered blood pressure
		Rapid, deep breathing
		Loss of consciousness

Emergency treatment	Glucose in rapidly absorbed form	Insulin Fluid and electrolyte replacement Sodium bicarbonate
Speed of response	Rapid	Slow

Prevention	Never interfere with normal mealtimes
	    of diabetic
	Never tell diabetic to fast without
	    seeking medical consult
	Have available a ready source of
	    glucose
	Careful observation for warning signs
		Never tell diabetic not to take
		    medication without medical consult
		Careful observation for warning signs

23. (pp. 617-628)

	Type 1 (IDDM)	**Type 2 (NIDDM)**
Percentage of individuals with DM	20%	80%
Age of onset	Preadolescent	Over 30
Speed of onset of symptoms	Acute	Insidious
Family history	Yes	Very strong
Body build	Thin	Obese
Presence of autoantibodies	Yes	No
Insulin receptor defects	No	Yes
Severity of manifestations	Acute	Mild

(cont'd)

	Type 1 (IDDM), cont'd	Type 2 (NIDDM), cont'd
Stability	More difficult	More stable
Frequency of complications	Frequent	Less common
Occurrence of ketoacidosis	Frequent	Less common
Frequency of hypoglycemia	Frequent	Less common
Treatment with insulin	Always	Less common
Treatment with oral hypoglycemics	No	Frequent

24. (p. 628, Fig. 25-10, p. 630) Hypoparathyroidism leads to hypocalcemia, which affects nerve and muscle function. It can lead to weak cardiac muscle contractions but increased excitability of nerves, leading to spontaneous contractions of skeletal muscle: twitching and spasms.
25. (p. 629; Fig. 25-10, p. 630) Hyperparathyroidism causes hypercalcemia, which leads to forceful cardiac contractions; osteoporosis due to excess bone demineralization; and increased predisposition to kidney stones.
26. (p. 631) excess growth hormone secretions from a pituitary adenoma in the adult
27. (pp. 631-632, Fig. 25-12)
    Manifestations include
      bones that become broader and heavier

soft tissues that grow, resulting in enlarged hands and feet
a thicker skull
changes in facial features
Complications include
  nerve and blood vessel compression in the skull
  carpal tunnel syndrome
  arthritis
  diabetes
  hypertension and cardiovascular disease
28. (pp. 633-634, Figs. 25-13, 25-14) A goiter is an enlargement of the thyroid gland that is often visible on the neck; it is caused by hypothyroidism (endemic goiter) and hyperthyroidism (toxic goiter).
29. (pp. 633-636, Table 25-5)

	Hyperthyroidism	Hypothyroidism
Forms	Graves' disease	Infant: cretinism Adult: myxedema

Etiology	Autoimmune: thyroid-stimulating antibodies
	Adenoma: thyroid or pituitary
	Toxic goiter
		Congenital:
		  Thyroid agenesis or dysgenesis
		  Lower TSH or T_3 and T_4
		Adult:
		  Autoimmune (Hashimoto's disease)
		  Surgical removal
		  Drugs

Serum T_3 and T_4 levels	High	Low
Metabolic rate	High	Low
Nervous system effects	Restlessness, anxiety, irritability Insomnia Tremors Impaired concentration	Child: severe mental retardation Decreased reflexes Fatigue, sluggishness Headache Slow intellectual functions Coma
Cardiovascular effects	Tachycardia Palpitations, arrhythmias Increased blood pressure Cardiomegaly Severe: angina pectoris, myocardial infarction	Bradycardia Decreased CO Decreased blood pressure

	Hyperthyroidism, cont'd	Hypothyroidism, cont'd
Respiratory effects	Hyperventilation Dyspnea	Hypoventilation
Skeletal effects	Increased resorption Advanced bone age Osteoporosis	Retarded bone age "Stubby hands"

Muscular effects	Increased tone leading to tremors and
	  twitching
	Diarrhea
		Decreased tone and reflexes
		Muscle weakness
		Decreased peristalsis leading to
		  constipation, flatulence, and
		  abdominal distention

Skin and hair	Increased sweating Flushed warm skin Soft nails Thin, silky hair	Pale; yellowish hue Cool Dry and rough Hair brittle and coarse Alopecia Loss of lateral third of eyebrows
Temperature tolerance	Increased body temperature Heat intolerance	Decreased body temperature Cold intolerance
Eyes	Exophthalmos Decreased blinking and eye movements "Lid lag"	Puffy
Body weight	Decreased with increased appetite	Increased with decreased appetite Edematous
Presence of goiter	With Graves'	With endemic goiter
Treatment	Antithyroid agents Radioactive iodine Thyroidectomy	Replacement therapy

30. (pp. 636-639, Figs. 25-16 to 25-18; Table 25-6)

	Cushing's Syndrome	Addison's Disease
Etiology	Adrenal tumor Glucocorticoids therapy Pituitary tumor Paraneoplastic syndrome	Autoimmune destruction Prolonged treatment with corticosteroids Infections: tuberculosis, fungi, cancer

Physical appearance	Round "moon face"
	Thinning of skin
	Purple striae
	Ecchymoses
	Cervical or supraclavicular fat pads—
	  "buffalo hump"
	Hirsutism
	Alopecia
	Protruding abdomen
		Hyperpigmentation of skin, particularly
		  in creases—also buccal mucosa and
		  tongue—"bronzing"

Fluid and electrolytes	Increased Na^+ and Cl^- Decreased K^+ Increased HCO_3^- and decreased H^+ Water retention resulting in edema	Decreased Na^+ and Cl^- Increased K^+ Increased H^+ and decreased HCO_3^- Dehydration

(cont'd)

Answer Key

	Cushing's Syndrome, cont'd	Addison's Disease, cont'd
Blood pressure	Increased	Decreased
Blood sugar	Increased	Normal or decreased ↓
Musculoskeletal effects	Atrophy Osteoporosis	Weakness
Inflammatory response	Decreased	Decreased
Immune response	Decreased	Decreased
Response to stress	Decreased	Decreased
Treatment	Surgery Palliative treatment: diuretics, antihypertensives, hypoglycemics or insulin antibiotics, etc.	Replacement therapy

31. (p. 638) Excessive glucocorticoids depress both inflammation and immunity, thereby impairing normal defenses. Antibacterial drugs are prescribed in an effort to prevent infection.
32. (pp. 617-641)
    i. Graves' disease: thyroid (T_3 and T_4) hypersecretion
    ii. gigantism: growth hormone hypersecretion as a child
    iii. myxedema: hyposecretion of thyroid hormones T_3 and T_4 as an adult
    iv. diabetes insipidus: hyposecretion of ADH
    v. acromegaly: growth hormone hypersecretion as an adult
    vi. Cushing's syndrome: hypersecretion of glucocorticoids
    vii. dwarfism: hyposecretion of growth hormone
    viii. diabetes mellitus: hyposecretion of insulin
    ix. Addison's disease: hyposecretion of mineralocorticoids, glucocorticoids and androgens
    x. cretinism: hyposecretion of thyroid hormones as a child
33. (pp. 617-641)
    i. hyperglycemia: diabetes mellitus, Cushing's, acromegaly
    ii. increased basal metabolic rate: hyperthyroidism
    iii. increased susceptibility to infection: diabetes mellitus, Addison's, Cushing's
    iv. intolerance to cold: hypothyroidism
    v. development of osteoporosis or decreased bone density: Cushing's hyperthyroidism, hyperparathyroidism
    vi. mental retardation: cretinism (hypothyroidism as child)
    vii. predisposition to renal calculi: hyperparathyroidism
    vii. hypotension: Addison's, hypothyroidism
    ix. impaired physical growth: hypothyroidism—cretinism, hyposecretion of growth hormone

    x. hyperpigmentation of the skin and oral mucosa: Addison's
    xi. an autoimmune disorder: diabetes mellitus type 1, hyperthyroidism—Graves', hypothyroidism—Hashimoto's
    xii. development of peripheral edema: inappropriate ADH syndrome, hypothyroidism—myxedema, Cushing's
    xiii. development of exophthalmos: hyperthyroidism—Graves'
    xiv. bradycardia: hypothyroidism
    xv. delayed clotting: Cushing's
    xvi. poor healing: Cushing's, hypothyroidism
    xvii. poor response to stress: Addison's, Cushing's, hyperthyroidism
    xviii. development or exacerbation of hypertension: diabetes mellitus, inappropriate ADH syndrome, hyperthyroidism, Cushing's
    xix. weight loss: diabetes mellitus, hyperthyroidism
    xx. presence of a goiter: hyperthyroidism (Graves'), hypothyroidism (endemic)
    xxi. enlarged hands and feet: acromegaly
    xxii. tachycardia and palpitations: hyperthyroidism
    xxiii. hyponatremia: inappropriate ADH syndrome, Addison's
    xxiv. hypocalcemia: hypoparathyroidism

CHAPTER 26

Musculoskeletal Disorders

1. (pp. 652-653, Fig. 26-4)
    i. compound: an open fracture—then the skin is broken; more damage to soft tissue
    ii. comminuted: multiple fracture lines and bone fragments
    iii. compression: when a bone is crushed or collapses into small pieces
    iv. greenstick: bone is only partially broken, shaft is bent, tearing the cortical bone on one side

v. impacted: one end of the bone is forced or telescoped into the adjacent bone

vi. oblique: fracture at an angle to the diaphysis of the bone

vii. pathological: fracture results from a weakness in bone structure; due to tumor or osteoporosis

viii. spiral: a break that angles around the bone; usually due to a twisting injury

ix transverse: a fracture across the bone

x. Colles': break in the distal radius at the wrist

2. (pp. 652-654; Fig. 26-5) Bleeding occurs and inflammation develops around the bone due to the soft tissue damage. A hematoma or clot forms in the medullary canal, under the periosteum. Necrosis occurs at the ends of the broken bone. The hematoma serves as a basis for fibrin network into which granulation tissue grows. Capillaries extend into tissue; phagocytic cells clean up debris. Fibroblasts (collagen) and chondroblasts (cartilage) migrate to the fibrin network. Bone ends become splinted by a procallus or fibrocartilaginous collar. Osteoblasts generate new bone, and callus is replaced, forming a bony callus. New bone is remodeled by osteoblastic and osteoclastic activity.

3. (pp. 654-655) Complications include muscle spasm causing abnormalities in the bone during the healing process, infections, ischemia, compartment syndrome, fat emboli, nerve damage, nonunion—failure to heal or malunion (deformity), and residual effects of fractures near a joint: osteoarthritis; stunted growth in children.

4. (pp. 655-656) Reduction of a fracture is the manipulation of the fracture to restore bones to their normal position and alignment. A closed reduction is done by exerting pressure and traction. An open reduction requires surgery; devices may be placed to fix the fragments.

5. (p. 656, Fig. 26-6) Dislocation is the separation of two bones at a joint with loss of contact between the articular surfaces. Subluxation is the partial displacement of bone with partial loss of contact between surfaces.

6. (p. 656) A sprain is a tear in a ligament. An avulsion occurs when a tendon or ligament is completely separated from its bony attachment.

7. (p. 658)
aging
decreased mobility or sedentary lifestyle
hormonal factors such as hyperparathyroidism, Cushing's syndrome
deficits of calcium, vitamin D or history of childhood deficits or malabsorption disorders
cigarette smoking
small, light bone structure
excessive caffeine intake

8. (p. 657) bones consisting of higher proportions of cancellous bone, such as vertebrae and the femoral neck

9. (p. 657) Bone resorption exceeds bone formation during the continuous process of bone remodeling, leading to thin, fragile bones.

10. (p. 658) Treatment includes dietary supplements, fluoride supplements, bisphosphonates, calcitonin and human parathyroid hormone, weight-bearing exercises, raloxifene, and possibly newer medications under investigation such as strontium ranelate; antibody that binds to osteoclasts.

11. (p. 658)

	Rickets	Osteomalcia	Paget's Disease
Etiology	Vitamin D deficiency in children due to diet or malabsorption	Vitamin D or calcium deficiency in adults	Idiopathic Unknown virus Genetic factors
Manifestations	Deformities—"bow legs" Decreased height	Soft bones Compression fractures	Pathologic fractures Compression fractures of vertebrae; kyphosis Compression of cranial nerves Cardiovascular disease and heart failure
Treatment	Supplements Treat malabsorption	Supplements	Supportive

12. (p. 658) long-term use of barbiturates (e.g., in treatment of epilepsy)

13. (p. 659) Osteosarcoma is a primary malignant neoplasm that usually develops in the metaphysis of the femur, tibia, or fibula in children or young adults, particularly males (Fig. 26-7). Chondrosarcomas are malignant tumors arising from cartilage and are more common in adults.

14. (p. 659, Fig. 26-8) The basic pathophysiology is the same in all types of muscular dystrophy. A metabolic defect, a deficit of dystrophin, a muscle cell membrane protein, leads to degeneration and necrosis of the cell. Skeletal muscle fibers are replaced by fat and fibrous connective tissue, leading to the hypertrophic appearance of the muscle.

15. (See Table 26-1, p. 660)

16. (p. 661) pain and stiffness affecting muscles, tendons, and surrounding soft tissues (not joints); other manifestations: sleep disturbances, depression, possibly irritable bowel syndrome, urinary symptoms

17. (p. 661) It is a degenerative processes. There is an increased incidence with age and excessive mechanical stress.

18. (pp. 661-665, Figs. 26-9 to 26-13)

	Osteoarthritis	Rheumatoid Arthritis
Etiology	Degenerative Primary: idiopathic Secondary: injury Genetic factor	Autoimmune Genetic factor
Predisposing factors	Age Obesity Any joint injury Familial tendency	Familial predisposition Females
Joints involved	Weight-bearing and those frequently injured—hips and knees, cervical and lumbar spine, distal interphalangeal, temporomandibular	Symmetrical involvement Small joints of hands and feet Wrists and ankles Temporomandibular
Pathophysiology	Damage of articular cartilage leads to interferes with movement resulting in further damage, exposure of endochondral bone and development of cysts and osteophytes that causes joint space narrowing Inflammation in surrounding soft tissue	Synovitis leads to pannus formation resulting in cartilage erosion, fibrosis, and finally ankylosis Muscle atrophy Development of malalignments, contractures, and deformities
Manifestations	Pain with use Limited movement Enlarged, hard joints Crepitus No systemic manifestations	Aching and stiffness Impaired mobility Deformities → functional losses
Extra-articular manifestations	None	Rheumatoid factor (RF) in blood Elevated ESR Low-grade fever, malaise, fatigue Subcutaneous nodules: pleura, heart valves, eyes
Treatment	NSAIDs Minimize stress on joint Ambulatory aids Orthotic devices Arthroplasty Joint replacement	Physiotherapy; ambulatory aids Occupational therapy: assistive devices NSAIDs, COX-2 inhibitors Glucocorticoids Immunosuppressants Gold salts Synovectomy Arthroplasty Joint replacement

19. (p. 665)
NSAIDs, COX-2 inhibitors
glucocorticoids
immunosuppressants
antimalarials
gold salts

20. (p. 666) The onset is usually more acute. Systemic effects are more marked, but rheumatoid nodules are absent. Large joints are frequently affected. Rheumatoid factor is not usually present. Other abnormal antibodies (e.g., ANA) may be present. The systemic form, Still's disease, develops with fever, rash, lymphadenopathy, and hepatomegaly, as well as joint involvement.

21. (p. 666, Fig, 26-14) deposits of uric acid and urate crystals in the joint that cause an acute inflammatory response

22. (p. 666) Gout is usually due to a metabolic abnormality, resulting in hyperuricemia. It often affects only single joint. It is more common in men over age

40. There is tophi formation, deposits of urate crystals.

23. (p. 667) Pathological changes include inflammation of the vertebral joints, fibrosis and calcification or fusion of the joints, inflammation that begins in the lower back at sacroiliac joints and progresses up spine, kyphosis, and osteoporosis; lung expansion may be limited at late stage due to calcification of the costovertebral joints.

24. (pp. 659-665).
   i. loss of articular cartilage; osteoarthritis, rheumatoid arthritis
   ii. development of tophi in soft tissue, bone, or both: gout
   iii. possible presence of an antibody against IgG in the serum: rheumatoid arthritis
   iv. classified as an autoimmune disease: rheumatoid arthritis
   v. presence of extra-articular (i.e., systemic) manifestations: rheumatoid arthritis, gout, ankylosing spondylitis
   vi. a sex-linked disorder: Duchenne's muscular dystrophy
   vii. may be treated with estrogen replacement therapy: osteoporosis
   viii. most commonly affects weight-bearing joints: osteoarthritis
   ix. incidence is highest in women between the ages of 20 and 50: fibromyalgia
   x. characterized by synovitis and pannus formation: rheumatoid arthritis
   xi. treatment may involve intra-articular injections of glucocorticoids: rheumatoid arthritis
   xii. may result in the development of kyphosis: osteoporosis, ankylosing spondylitis
   xiii. may be accompanied by ocular complications such as uveitis: rheumatoid arthritis, ankylosing spondylitis
   xiv. affects joints in hands and feet: rheumatoid arthritis
   xv. characterized by elevated serum uric acid levels: gout
   xvi. development of ankylosis or joint fusion over time: rheumatoid arthritis, ankylosing spondylitis
   xvii. treated with NSAIDs: osteoarthritis, rheumatoid arthritis, gout, ankylosing spondylitis
   xviii. immunosuppressants sometimes prescribed during exacerbations: rheumatoid arthritis
   xix. characterized by the development of osteophytes: osteoarthritis
   xx. primary involvement occurs in the sacroiliac and intervertebral joints: ankylosing spondylitis
   xxi. characterized by compression fractures of the vertebral bodies: osteoporosis
   xxii. crepitus is often present: osteoarthritis
   xxiii. treated with biphosphonates: osteoporosis

CHAPTER 27

Skin Disorders

1. (pp. 677-689)

Condition	Etiology	Treatment
Scleroderma	Unknown; may be local or systemic	NSAIDs and glucocorticoids
Kaposi's sarcoma	Rare skin cancer that occurs in immunosuppressed patients (especially AIDS)	Radiation and chemotherapy
Tinea	Fungal infections of various parts of the body caused by various species of Trichophyton	Oral antifungal agents such as griseofulvin Topical antifungal agents: griseofulvin; tolnaftate or ketoconazole
Atopic dermatitis	Type 1 hypersensitivity, with inherited tendency or genetic component	Topical glucocorticoids
Pemphigus	Autoimmune disorder	Systemic glucocorticoids
Herpes zoster	Varicella zoster virus	Antiviral medications for symptoms; e.g., acyclovir
Herpes simples	HSV-1	Topical acyclovir
Verrucae	Human papillomaviruses	Topical medications; laser and cryotherapy

(cont'd)

Condition, cont'd	Etiology, cont'd	Treatment, cont'd
Urticaria	Type 1 hypersensitivity to certain ingested substances; e.g., shellfish	Topical antihistamines or topical glucocorticoids
Psoriasis	Unknown; familial tendency	Glucocorticoids; tar preparations, and methotrexate when severe
Scabies	Mite infection by *Sarcoptes* scabiei	Topical treatment with lindane
Lichen planus	Unknown inflammatory condition of skin and mucous membranes	Topical glucocorticoids
Impetigo	*Staphylococcus aureus*	Topical and systemic antimicrobials
Cellulitis	Infection of dermis and subcutaneous tissue, secondary to an injury; *S. aureus*	Systemic antimicrobials; local compression and analgesics
Necrotizing fasciitis	Group A β-hemolytic streptococcus	Antimicrobials, fluid replacement, excision of all infected tissue and amputation if necessary

2. (pp. 686-688):
   i. those with excessive, cumulative sun (UV) exposure
   ii. those with malignant melanoma; genetic predisposition; hormonal factors; UV radiation (sunlight)
   iii. immunosuppressed patients; e.g., people with AIDS

3. (Table 27-1, p. 676) answer to crossword puzzle

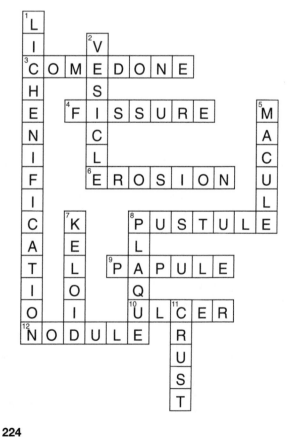

4. (pp. 674-688)
   i. Kaposi's sarcoma
   ii. urticaria
   iii. pemphigus
   iv. herpes zoster
   v. scabies
   vi. herpes simplex 1
   vii. verrucae
   viii. mycoses
   ix. atopic dermatitis
   x. scleroderma

CHAPTER 28

Reproductive System Disorders

1. (pp. 693, 703)
males: changes in sperm or semen, hormonal abnormalities, physical obstruction of the sperm passage
females: hormonal imbalances resulting from altered function of hypothalamus, anterior pituitary, or ovaries, structural abnormalities, obstruction of fallopian tubes, abnormal vaginal pH, cigarette smoking

2. (pp. 693-695)
   i. hypospadias: urethral opening on the ventral surface of the penis
   ii. epispadias: urethral opening on the dorsal surface of the penis
   iii. cryptorchidism: undescended testes (Fig. 28-2)
   iv. hydrocele: excessive fluid collects between the layers of the tunica vaginalis (Fig. 28-3)
   v. spermatocele: cyst containing fluid and sperm that develops between the testes and the epididymis
   vi. varicocele: dilated vein in the spermatic cord (Fig. 28-3)

3. (p. 696) young men in association with urinary tract infections, older men with benign prostatic hypertrophy, sexually transmitted diseases, instrumentation such as catheterization

4. (p. 696) *Escherichia coli*

5. (p. 696)
dysuria
urinary frequency
urgency
low back pain or lower abdominal discomfort
severe inflammation may cause:
    decreased urinary stream
    hesitancy in initiating urination
    incomplete bladder emptying
    nocturia

6. (p. 696) hyperplasia of the prostatic tissue with formation of nodules surrounding the urethra, compression of the urethra and variable degrees of urinary obstruction

7. (pp. 696-697, Fig. 28-5) incomplete bladder emptying due to obstruction leads to frequent infections, continued obstruction leads to distended bladder, dilated ureters, hydronephrosis, and possible renal damage

8. (p. 697) hesitancy, dribbling, decreased force of the urinary stream, frequency, nocturia, recurrent infections

9. (pp. 697-698) Cause has not been determined. Genetic and hormonal factors appear to be involved. It is common in men of North American and northern European descent. There is a higher incidence in the black population.

10. (p. 698) Warning signs include hard nodule in the periphery of the gland on rectal exam, elevated prostate specific antigen (not diagnostic, also occurs with benign prostatic hypertrophy), and signs of urinary obstruction.

11. (pp. 697-698, Fig. 28-6) metastasis to bone: spine, pelvis, ribs, and femur

12. (p. 698) PSA, or prostate specific antigen

13. (p. 698) Removal of androgen-sensitive tumors may be suggested to reduce hormonal effects.

14. (p. 699) Risk factors include familial incidence, cryptorchidism, infection, and trauma.

15. (p. 699) Manifestations include hard, painless, usually unilateral mass; enlarged or "heavy" testes; dull aching pain in the lower abdomen; and gynecomastia.

16. (p. 699) Treatment includes a combination of surgery, radiation, and chemotherapy.

17. (pp. 704-705, Fig. 28-10)
    i. anteflexion: uterus bent forward over the bladder
    ii. retroflexion: uterus is flexed posteriorly
    iii. cystocele urinary bladder bulges into vagina
    iv. rectocele: rectum bulges into vagina
    v. uterine prolapse: uterus descent into the vagina to varying degrees
    vi. dysmenorrhea: painful menses
    vii. amenorrhea: no menses

    viii. dyspareunia: painful intercourse

18. (p. 706, Fig. 28-11) The presence of endometrial tissue outside of the uterus on structures such as the ovaries, ligaments, or colon.

19. (p. 706, Fig. 28-11) Ectopic endometrium responds to cyclic hormonal changes just as normal uterus; no exit point for shed tissue and blood, causes local inflammation and pain, recurring with each menstrual cycle. Fibrous tissue may cause adhesions and obstruction of involved structures such as urinary bladder and colon and ovary (infertility).

20. (p. 707) dysmenorrhea

21. (p. 707) Treatment involves hormonal suppression of endometrial tissue and surgical removal of ectopic tissue.

22. (p. 707) Predisposing factors include antimicrobial therapy for an unrelated bacterial infection, immunodeficiency states, increased glycogen or glucose in secretions, use of oral contraceptives, and diabetes mellitus.

23. (p. 707)
red and swollen pruritic mucous membranes
thick, white, curd-like discharge
white patches adhering to the vaginal wall
dysuria
dyspareunia

24. (p. 707) an infection of the reproductive tract, particularly the fallopian tubes and ovaries; includes cervicitis, endometritis, salpingitis, and oophoritis

25. (pp. 708-709) Predisposing factors for PID include sexually transmitted disease, prior episode of vaginitis or cervicitis, insertion of an IUD or other instrument, septicemia, or peritoneal infections.

26. (pp. 707-708, Fig. 28-12)
vaginitis or cervicitis of polymicrobial etiology
ascending inflammation and infection from uterus into fallopian tubes, causing edema and obstruction
exudate contaminates ovary and surrounding tissue
peritonitis may develop, with pelvic abscess formation
potential septicemia
adhesions and strictures common sequelae, leading to infertility or ectopic pregnancy, as well as affecting surrounding structures such as the colon

27. (p. 709)
lower abdominal pain, which may be sudden and severe or gradually increasing in intensity
steady pain that increases with walking
tenderness
purulent discharge
dysuria
fever and leukocytosis
abdominal distention and rigidity indicate peritonitis

28. (p. 708) Complications if untreated include pelvic abscess, septicemia, death, adhesions, and strictures of surrounding tissues: infertility or ectopic pregnancy.

29. (p. 709) aggressive antimicrobial therapy

Answer Key

30. (p. 713) Increased use of Pap smear for screening has had two results:

Early detection allows for effective treatment at early stage, improving prognosis and survival.

Early detection while cancer is still in situ; more cases are detected early in a younger population.

31. (p. 714) Individuals at high risk include those with multiple sexual partners, those with promiscuous partners, early sexual intercourse in teen years, a history of STDs, and environmental factors such as smoking cigarettes.

32. (p. 713, Fig. 28-15)

cervical dysplasia—mild

cervical dysplasia—severe

malignant neoplasm

carcinoma in situ

invasive carcinoma

33. (p. 714)

asymptomatic early but detectable by Pap smear

slight bleeding or watery discharge

anemia or weight loss

34. (p. 714) Biopsy confirms the diagnosis. Surgery combined with radiation is the recommended treatment.

35. (p. 715) Individuals at high risk include those with a history of increased estrogen levels, postmenopausal women who have taken exogenous estrogen, infertile women, those who took sequential oral contraceptives early, obese women, those with diabetes, and those with hypertension.

36. (p. 715)

endometrial hyperplasia of the glandular epithelium (d/t excessive estrogen stimulation)

slow growth and infiltration of uterine wall

continued growth results in tumor mass filling the interior of the uterus and infiltrating and extending through the wall into surrounding structures

grading and staging determined by degree of cell differentiation/undifferentiation (grade) and extent of spread (stage)

37. (p. 715) Manifestations include painless vaginal bleeding or spotting (early sign), palpable mass, discomfort or pressure in the lower abdomen, and bleeding following intercourse (late sign).

38. (pp. 712, 714-715) surgery and radiation therapy

39. (p. 712) Risk factors include being over the age of 50, having a genetic predisposition, familial occurrence, hormonal influences especially exposure to high estrogen levels, long menstrual cycles, and delay in first pregnancy. Exogenous estrogen in oral contraceptives or postmenopausal supplements as a cause is controversial. Other factors include fibrocystic disease, prior carcinoma in the uterus or other breast, and radiation of the chest.

40. (p. 712)

majority arise from malignant transformation of ductal epithelial cells

local infiltration of surrounding tissues and adherence to skin causing dimpling

spread to nearby axillary lymph nodes early

widespread dissemination follows quickly including metastases to lung, brain, bond, and liver

41. (p. 712) Manifestations include

single small, hard, painless nodule in the breast; freely moveable in early stages

dimpling of the skin, fixation of the nodule to the skin, retraction of or discharge from the nipples, and change in breast contour

42. (p. 712) Therapeutic interventions include surgical removal of the tumor with minimal tissue loss or a more radical mastectomy combined with radiation and chemotherapy. Surgical of some lymph nodes is usually warranted. The ovaries are removed if the tumor is responsive to hormones.

43. (p. 713) Early detection measures include breast self-examination regularly for all women older than 20 and mammography, especially if family history warrants, and routinely after age 40.

44. (See Table 28-1, p. 717)